2-WEEK TURNAROUND DIET
Cookbook

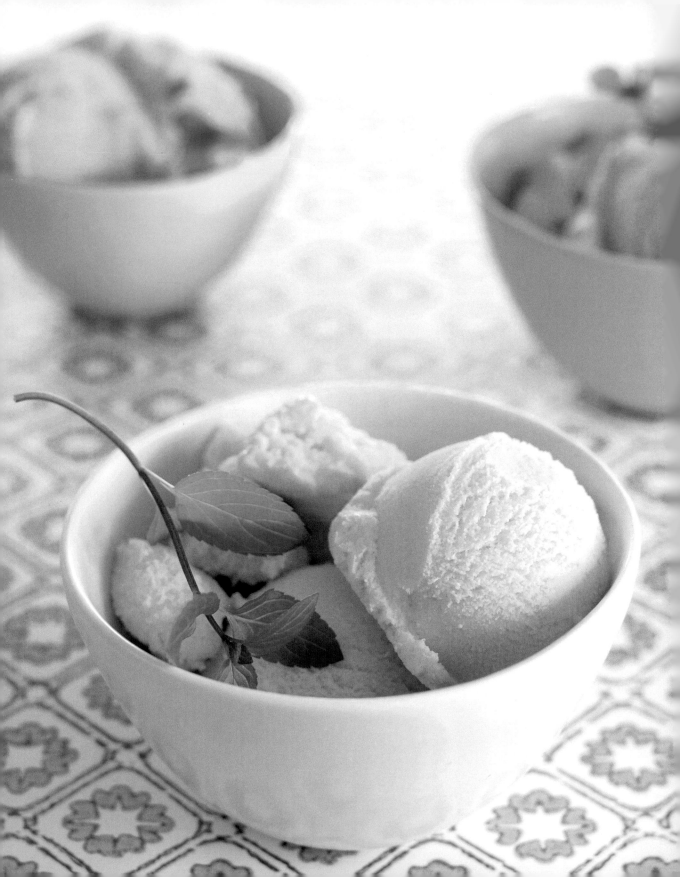

2-WEEK TURNAROUND™ DIET
Cookbook

Jump-start weight loss
with more than 150 delicious meals

HEATHER K. JONES, RD,
WITH CHRIS FREYTAG,
CONTRIBUTING EDITOR OF
Prevention.

RODALE

contents

acknowledgments

BOOKS THIS MEATY COME TOGETHER WITH THE HELP OF MANY PEOPLE. We'd like to thank the following for all of their efforts in helping to pull the delicious meals and important nutritional information together. Our appreciation goes to Anne Egan, Paul Piccuito, Sidra Forman, Kathy Hanuschak, Juhie Bhatia, and Kate Winne.

We'd also like to thank the team at Rodale and at *Prevention*, especially Andrea Au Levitt, Marielle Messing, Jill Armus, Carol Angstadt, Toby Fox, Shana Sobel, Sandy Freeman, Chris Krogermeier, Brooke Myers, Janelle Wagner, and Lois Hazel. We are thrilled to have had JoAnn Brader and her team in the Rodale Test Kitchen evaluate the recipes, ensuring they will work every time.

—Heather K. Jones and Chris Freytag

foreword

The *2-Week Total Body Turnaround* was meant to be intense—a kick in the butt, a mental challenge, a contest to keep you going for 14 days. It was designed to give you the skills and tools you need to get started on the road toward better health. I believe that more than half the battle of weight loss is finding the motivation to get started and gaining the knowledge to believe you are doing it "right" and should persevere.

I also believe that knowledge is power and what you don't know *can* hurt you. Making healthy eating choices is about understanding food and how it works within your body. I'm a 44-year-old working mom with three teenagers and a very hectic schedule. I understand how challenging it can be to get started on an exercise and eating plan when your calendar is overbooked and your to-do list is a few inches long.

That's why Heather K. Jones, a top-notch registered dietitian and weight loss consultant, and I have created the *2-Week Turnaround Diet Cookbook*. Keeping today's busy lifestyles in mind, we designed this easy-to-follow eating plan and its 160 simple yet delicious recipes.

I have always said, "You are what you eat." The 2-Week Turnaround is as much about the nutrition side of the equation as it is about the physical and mental side. The foods you eat greatly affect your mood, appearance, and weight loss efforts. That's why the recipes in this book use whole foods (what I call "clean" eating), such as fresh fruits and vegetables, low-fat or fat-free dairy, whole grains or grain alternatives, lean meats, poultry, and fish. The meals avoid using preservatives, additives, processed sugars, and general "junk food" as much as possible, while still maintaining flavor for you and your family.

I know it isn't always easy, and believe me, I have my moments when I struggle with food choices. But new behavior is learned by repetition. So by dedicating yourself to 2 weeks of focused and thoughtful eating and exercise, you are giving yourself the chance to change and the chance to form new habits. As the saying goes, "Try it, you may like it." I have often had clients tell me there is no way their kids will eat flaxseed, only to find that my amazing homemade Peanut Butter and Chocolate Energy Bars (recipe on page 235) are devoured every time.

So keep an open mind, try new foods, and take this journey to a healthier lifestyle with a positive attitude. I am proud of you for taking the first step. And after you finish the 14 days, I hope you can throw up your hands with confidence and declare, "If I can do 2 weeks, I can do anything!"

—Chris Freytag

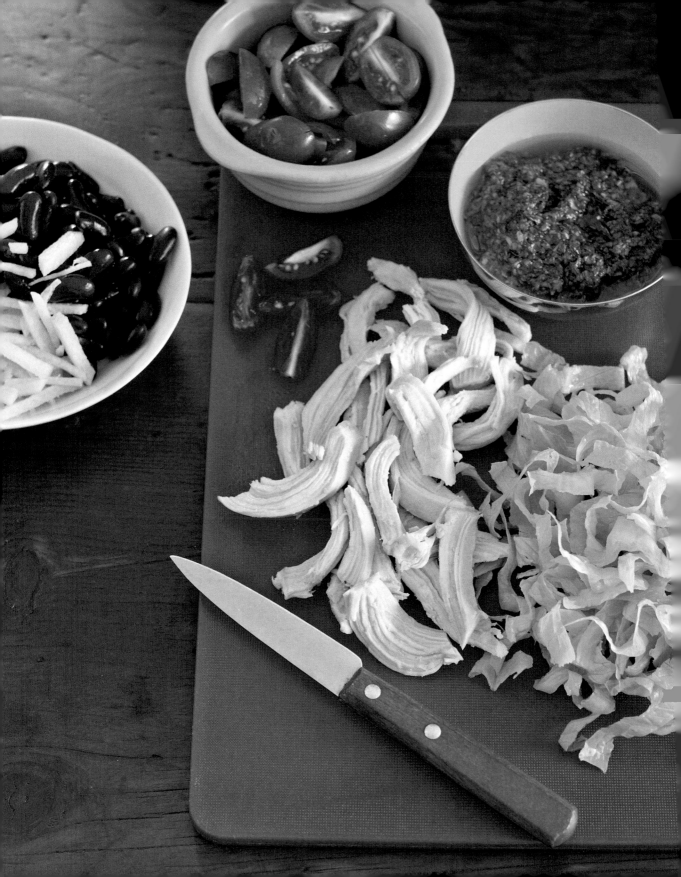

introduction

Turnaround Time

Two weeks may not seem like a long time, but it's really all the time you need to turn your health habits around. It's true! In just 14 days you can make the necessary changes to slim your waistline and lay the foundation for health-boosting eating behaviors that last. And you won't have to kill yourself in the process, I promise. I'm a registered dietitian, health advocate, weight loss counselor, and health journalist who has spent the last decade helping people who struggle with weight management. I spent seven of those years working for the *Nutrition Action Healthletter*, the nation's largest-circulation health newsletter. I'm the author of *What's Your Diet Type?* and *The Grocery Cart Makeover* and a nutrition consultant for *The Best Life Diet* by Bob Greene, Oprah's personal fitness trainer. In my experience, 14 days is all the time you need to make a major change in your diet.

Those of you who have already done Chris Freytag's wonderful *2-Week Total Body Turnaround* exercise program, which works hand in hand with this book, have hopefully already experienced this success for yourself. Now be prepared to be amazed again. We've created the *2-Week Turnaround Diet Cookbook* to round out the exercise program and to further maximize your results over the next 2 weeks. Healthy living is really a combination of being physically active, eating smart, and maintaining mental fitness; between these two books you'll learn how to improve all three for the total health package.

The tips, skills, and tools you'll acquire over the next 14 days will not only kick off your healthy living regimen, but they'll also instill eating and exercise habits that can last a lifetime. For 2 weeks, I'll guide you through the plan, suggesting what to eat, and how to stay motivated. But don't get frightened: It will be real work, but it will also be worth it. Your reward? You'll look and feel your best.

The Workout Plan

Chris Freytag created the *2-Week Total Body Turnaround* program in response to requests from clients she met during more than 17 years working in the health and fitness industry as a personal trainer and coach, group fitness instructor, weight management consultant, and motivational speaker. Women told her they needed an exercise program that could realistically fit into their busy schedules. Not only that, they wanted the plan to yield fast results and provide the tools and motivation to stick with it in the long run.

So Chris joined forces with Alyssa Shaffer and *Prevention* magazine to design a research-based, reader-tested, 2-week exercise program that helps you blast calories, boost metabolism, drop inches everywhere—especially in the dreaded belly area—and permanently alter your fitness-related thinking. This program will jump-start weight loss for all women, whether you've fallen off the exercise wagon or are getting in shape for the first time in your life. Regardless of why you've turned to the 2-Week Turnaround workout plan, you'll feel your energy levels skyrocket, your endurance increase, and newfound confidence enter your step.

The best part about this exercise program is that it doesn't require you to spend hours a day working out in the gym. The regimen has been created with your hectic life in mind, so you'll build muscle, lose fat, and rev up your metabolism in just 1 hour a day. If that seems like a lot of time for you, just remember it's only for 2 weeks. The program is a perfect mix of strength-building exercises and fat- and calorie-burning cardio, so you'll simultaneously tone up and lose weight. On each of the 14 days, you'll follow a clearly laid-out plan that includes 30 minutes of Chris's signature strength-training exercises, proven to be among the most effective to firm up all major muscle groups. You'll alternate between doing upper-body plus core exercises, lower-body plus core ones, and total-body moves with each workout. For the cardio part of the plan, you'll spend 30 minutes daily doing the walking program. Rest assured, you'll also get some downtime. Each week you'll have 1 day of active rest and recovery so you can recuperate.

After 2 weeks on this plan, you're sure to see results. The program helped the test panel of 30 women, who were all in different places in their lives. In just 14 days, these women lost an average of nearly 6 pounds and 10½ inches—and some women lost as much as 12 pounds and a total of more than 22 inches! Every one of the women said that thanks to the plan, her energy levels soared, her sleep improved, and she felt stronger and healthier overall. The program also improved their mental health, as all the women felt more confident after seeing what they could accomplish. Since the book came out in 2009, it has gone on to help thousands of other women who have dropped dress sizes and boosted their overall health, and who now feel fabulous.

Eating Right for Life

When it comes to weight loss and general health, watching what you eat is just as important as the exercises you do. The foods you choose can optimize your workouts, help you shed pounds quicker, and further boost your energy levels and metabolism. That's why throughout the 2-Week Total Body Turnaround, Chris provided smart eating tips and a sample eating plan that was integrated with the workout program.

But as people embarked on the exercise plan, Chris started to get requests for further advice on healthy eating basics, more tasty recipes, and additional smart-eating tips and tricks. In response to the demand, Chris teamed up with me, and together we created the *2-Week Turnaround Diet Cookbook* to help you maximize the smart-eating part of the healthy lifestyle equation. This easy-to-follow eating plan meshes perfectly with the exercise program, providing 14 days of healthful, nutrient-dense menus to accompany each day that you'll be working out. As you read this book, you'll notice that the daily menu includes a nutritious breakfast, lunch, and dinner, as well as two snacks.

You'll be happy to know that this is not a starvation diet that leaves your stomach growling all day long or a time-consuming eating plan. We designed this diet keeping your jam-packed schedule and love of food in mind. So not only do we provide 14 days of menus, but you'll also find 160 delicious and nutritionally balanced recipes—along with dozens of ideas for super-quick meals you can throw together when you're short on time. And you can mix and match the recipes to create meal plans that best suit your tastes and needs if the sample menus don't work for you. The combination of nutrients provided in these meals—plus the tips we offer on meal timing—will help you feel satisfied all day long, as well as provide your body with optimum fuel for the physical activity you'll be doing almost daily. Through the wide variety of foods you'll be consuming on this diet, your body will have everything it needs for enhanced health and fitness. Also, because nutrient-dense foods have a high nutrient-to-calorie ratio (meaning they're rich in nutrients when compared to their calorie content), you'll be eating heartier portions of food while still taking in fewer calories. So trust me, you'll never be hungry on this plan!

Ultimately, though, like the workout plan, this eating plan has been designed to aid you in the long run. We've worked hard to provide you with all the tools you need to not only eat right for 2 weeks, but ideally for the rest of your life. So as you flip through these pages, you'll also find detailed information on the fundamentals of food, sample menus, and tips to cope with diet obstacles. The *2-Week Turnaround Diet Cookbook* presents you with a whole new way of eating, one that can be continually modified and adapted to suit your needs, so you see permanent results.

Think of both of these books as working together to be your guides to total fitness, healthy eating, and continued motivation for the long haul. As Chris tells her clients, "Motivation gets you started; habit keeps you going." Are you ready to jump in?

—*Heather K. Jones, RD*

EAT YOUR WAY TO
HEALTH

i f you're familiar with the *2-Week Total Body Turnaround* exercise program, you're already on the road to total fitness. But being active is only one part of the healthy living equation. Your diet is just as important.

The foods you choose to eat can maximize your workouts; they can also help you lose weight faster, increase your energy, boost your metabolism, and improve your overall health. In fact, what you use as fuel during these 2 weeks will make a big difference in your overall results. If you pay close attention to what you put into your body, you'll look and feel your best.

Eating your way to health is easy, but deciding what to eat, when to eat, and how to eat it can be more challenging. That's why we lay out the basics of healthy eating for you, provide 160 balanced and delicious recipes, and have created an easy-to-follow and flexible 2-week meal plan. The *2-Week Turnaround Diet Cookbook* is actually designed to mesh perfectly with the exercises you'll be doing, so your body will be fully fueled for physical activity each and every day. This nutrient-dense diet is loaded with a wide variety of healthy and delicious foods to ensure that your body gets exactly what it needs to work at an optimum level. And when every system in your body is working at an optimum level, your metabolism and ability to lose weight improve significantly.

We'll also provide tips and tricks to stay on the healthy eating track even after these 2 weeks are over, so you can form new habits that stick. Unlike other diets—I realize the word *diet* scares off many women!—this eating plan is designed for the long haul. It provides real opportunities to change, as you'll be examining your current food habits and then laying the foundation for healthier ones. This is not some fad diet that will lead to only temporary weight loss; it's a whole new way of eating. Once you get started, you'll see—it really is that easy. You only need 2 weeks to form healthy eating habits that last a lifetime.

"ALL GLORY COMES FROM DARING TO BEGIN."

—Eugene F. Ware

Eat Well

As you make your way through the *2-Week Turnaround Diet Cookbook*, one word should come to mind: flexibility. This do-it-yourself eating plan allows you to decide what to eat, based on some simple guidelines. And the 160 easy-to-follow and mouthwatering recipes in this book are varied enough to fit everyone's palette and budget.

This is a customized eating plan, which means you can mix and match the nutrient-packed food choices until you have a selection of menus that fit your tastes. For people who like structure, we provide suggested menus for the full 14 days. This includes three meals and two snacks a day. Each day of workouts from the *2-Week Total Body Turnaround* book is accompanied by a set of meals in this book. Don't like a recipe? No problem. You're free to swap out recipes for ones you like better. I want you to enjoy what you're eating; otherwise, it's unlikely that you'll stick to this eating plan for 2 weeks, much less a lifetime. Once you get the hang of how to combine the different food groups, you'll quickly realize that the possibilities for healthy eating are endless. For those of you who want complete freedom when planning your meals, you can choose from the many recipes to create your own meal plan for each day of the exercise program. It's really that simple.

Regardless of which recipes you pick, you'll find that each one is nutrient dense, well balanced, and very satisfying. The recipes have been created to provide the nutrients necessary to maximize your health and your workouts. You'll find a sensible mix of "good" carbohydrates, lean protein, and "good" fats, as well as foods that are high in fiber. This mix ensures stable blood-sugar and energy levels, and wards off cravings. Your goal is 1,600 calories a day, made up of carbs (about 45 percent of your daily calories), fat (about 25 percent), and protein (30 percent). You'll eat three healthy meals (at about 400 calories each) and two satisfying snacks (about 200 calories each). *Note:* For men on this plan, the total calorie count is 2,000, with three healthy meals (still at about 400 calories) and two snacks (at about 400 calories). Just as important as sticking to this nutrient-dense, satisfying eating plan is making eating whole foods a habit. Healthy foods, as Chris calls them, are whole and minimally processed foods, such as whole grains (like brown rice, quinoa, and oats), fresh fruits and vegetables, low-fat or fat-free dairy, lean meats, poultry, and fish. Eliminating as many of the preservatives, additives, processed sugars, and general junk from your diet as possible will keep your body in top condition. So it's time to clear your kitchen of any processed and junk foods, as none of them make the cut in this eating plan. Remember, this is a diet to stick to even after these 2 weeks are over, so start making a habit of replacing unhealthy food options with whole, healthful ones.

Eat Often

It's not only vital to focus on what you eat, but also when you eat. You want to be consuming food at regular intervals—five times a day—so you never allow yourself to get too hungry. We leave the exact timing of your meals up to you, but you must eat a healthy breakfast, lunch, and dinner (plus two snacks) every day to maximize your workouts. The goal is to eat every 3 to 4 hours so your blood-sugar levels don't dip too low. Once your glucose levels drop, cravings will kick in and suddenly anything in sight will start to look delicious.

Eating more often, on the other hand, may help you ward off cravings and lose weight. How? When you eat large meals with many hours in between, you train your metabolism to slow down. But having a small meal or snack every 3 to 4 hours keeps your metabolism going, so you burn more calories over the course of a day. Studies have also shown that people who snack between meals eat less at mealtime.[1, 2] Eating more frequently may help keep you feeling full and encourage you to eat more earlier in the day, which gives you more time to burn off calories. Additionally, snacking seems to be associated with a lower risk of heart disease, due to lower levels of both total and "bad" LDL cholesterol.[3]

Ultimately, when you choose to eat your snacks is up to you. Some people prefer to have a snack midmorning and then again after lunch to hold them over until dinner; others want something late at night. (Though I usually recommend avoiding late-night snacking, as it often turns into late-night bingeing and dessert overdose.) If you really want snack time to be in sync with your workouts, though, some times are better than others. There are ways to coordinate your snacks (and even your meals) to make the most of your exercise routine.

Timing Is Everything

One of the best times for your snack is about an hour before you work out. Fueling up with a small, energy-boosting snack, as well as some fluids, before your workout will not only keep you from feeling hungry, it will also maintain your blood-sugar levels and fight off fatigue during exercise.[4] However, if you've had a balanced meal within 2 hours of starting your workout, you shouldn't need to snack beforehand.

If you want to further maximize the results of the exercise program, keep in mind that what you eat during the hour after your workout is particularly important for building muscle and replenishing energy sources.

This period, known as the glycogen window, is when the muscles are better able to soak up nutrients and when glycogen (your stored form of energy) is replaced most efficiently. So try to have a muscle-building, protein-rich meal or snack during the hour after you work out as well.[5] This may be especially true for women, who may need protein after resistance training.[6] The snacks on this plan all contain dairy—and dairy foods are excellent sources of high-quality proteins. It's important that you reach for a savory snack, such as White Bean Dip (page 217), to keep blood sugar consistent and prevent energy crashes. Check out Chapter 2 (page 14) for details on why dairy foods are great for losing weight.

Spend More Time Eating

Another part of the healthy eating puzzle, in addition to changing what and when you eat, is looking at how you eat. Getting rid of old food behaviors that stand between you and a healthier life is key. The unfortunate reality is that for most of us there are constant obstacles to staying on the healthy eating track, whether it's fast food, meals on the go, binge eating, or overeating. I call these scenarios diet dilemmas. The challenges differ for each of us. For some people the dilemma is that pint of ice cream that calls their name when they're feeling down. For others it's having a hectic schedule that leaves little time to eat anything other than fast food. Some women beat themselves up for the slightest deviation from their diets or exercise plans, and then only unhealthy foods can provide consolation. Whether it's a bad food habit or a barrier to healthy eating, these diet dilemmas are real and present themselves to many of us each and every day.

While each diet dilemma has its own solution, a vital part of healthy eating is being conscious or mindful of what you eat. This means paying attention to what you're putting into your body and how it can impact your health and your waistline. The first step to mindful eating is to eat only when you're actually physically hungry, instead of turning to food when you're bored, stressed, sad, or when some other emotion hits. Not sure of the difference? There are some signs you can use to distinguish between physical hunger and emotional eating, stress eating, eating from boredom, or timed eating. Here are some differences between physical hunger and emotional hunger to keep in mind:

- Physical hunger is gradual (think stomach growling), while emotional hunger is abrupt (suddenly you're starving).

- When you're physically hungry, you are open to many different foods, whereas with emotional hunger your craving is usually for a specific food.

- There's usually no guilt or shame associated with physical hunger, while guilt often accompanies emotional hunger.

- When you're physically hungry, you usually stop eating when you're full, but with emotional hunger, you often don't notice or stop eating when you're full.

In addition to eating only when you're truly hungry, there are many other ways to be mindful of what you eat. Eat slowly, for instance, so you're actually tasting and enjoying what you eat, and stop eating when you're full. Don't eat on the go or in the car, and try to eat without any distractions (yes, this means not in front of the TV or the computer), as you're more likely to eat mindlessly in these scenarios.

These pointers are just the tip of the iceberg. Throughout this book, we'll present you with common diet pitfalls—from emotional eating to negative self-talk to handling food pushers—and then offer simple solutions to overcome these obstacles. Part of changing a harmful eating behavior is to understand why you do it and then how to get over it. By following these simple tips, you'll be well on your way to changing how you eat and forming a lifetime of healthy eating behaviors.

The Food–Body Connection

Closely following this eating plan—from what you eat to how you eat it—will not only boost your health, it will also prime you to gain the greatest benefit from your 2-Week Total Body Turnaround workouts. You'll feel better and see those pounds drop more quickly. Nothing works better to motivate you to stick to a plan for life than seeing fast results.

Here's how this eating plan works hand in hand with the exercise plan to maximize results:

- **SPEEDS WEIGHT LOSS**: You'll see those pounds melt off faster when you follow this eating plan, as it contains just the right number of nutrient-dense calories—enough calories to provide energy for your workouts, but not enough to cause you to store fat. Losing weight boils down to a very simple equation: calories in versus calories out. It's not about gimmicks or fads; it's just basic arithmetic. If you burn more calories than you eat, then you lose weight. But if you eat more than you burn, you'll gain weight. For instance, if you eat 1,600 calories—as in our eating plan—but burn 2,000, then you'll start to see that waistline shrink. Essentially, you need to create an energy deficit to truly lose weight, and you can do this by eating fewer calories or increasing the number of calories you burn through physical activity. And between our eating and exercise plans, you'll quickly burn calories.[7] Also, because this eating plan contains 1,600 calories worth of nutrient-packed foods, instead of 1,600 calories worth of empty-calorie foods (like cookies, chips, or candy), you're going to feel and look your best, and you're going to feel fuller. In fact, you'll never feel deprived or hungry on this plan because it includes about 25 grams of fiber per day—and fiber fills you up without adding calories. This can help you drop those pounds even faster.

INCREASES ENERGY: When you eat the right combination of foods, you'll feel your energy levels soar. Each nutrient-dense recipe gives you more than enough fuel to complete the exercise plan each day. How? Our meals have the perfect balance of carbs, protein, and fat to keep your blood-sugar levels stable, which not only wards off fatigue but will boost your energy levels in a sustained way. Carbs are key to providing energy when you work out,[8] so this meal plan is designed to maintain appropriate carbohydrate levels, with recipes that focus on nutrient-dense whole grains and fiber. If you also take advantage of snack timing (see page 3), having a snack 1 hour before your workout will further boost your energy levels while you exercise.

BOOSTS METABOLISM: This eating plan will boost your metabolism, which helps you lose weight in many different ways. By eating frequently, every 3 to 4 hours, you'll maintain your metabolism so that you can burn calories over the course of the day. If you leave lots of time between your meals, you actually start to train your metabolism to slow down.[9] Protein has also been shown to have a slight metabolism-boosting effect. Why? Because it takes our bodies about three times more energy—which means more burned calories—to digest protein than it does to digest carbs or fat.[10] So to help raise your metabolism on this eating plan, 30 percent of your total daily calories will come from lean protein. The diet also focuses on fiber and on complex carbs, which have less of an impact on insulin levels and discourage the metabolism from slowing down. Throughout the book we will highlight other foods and minerals that can jump-start your metabolism, such as calcium, grapefruit, and green tea.

BUILDS MUSCLE: Protein is crucial for building and repairing muscle fibers. Since you will be spending the next 2 weeks toning and sculpting your muscles, you'll want to make sure you have enough protein to let your muscles do their job. Not only that, but eating one of our nutrient-dense snacks or meals during the hour after you work out will also help you build muscle. All of our snacks include a serving of dairy, and since dairy foods are great sources of high-quality protein, they provide what you need to build and repair your muscles.

Get Ready

Now that you have an idea of what to expect over the next 2 weeks, you're ready to dive in! In the next chapter, we'll explore the specific foods you will—and won't—find in the *2-Week Turnaround Diet Cookbook*, and why these foods will boost your health and help you lose weight. We'll give you all the tools you need to create your own delicious eating plan, which will complement the exercise plan. By the end of the 2 weeks, you'll be an expert on healthy eating!

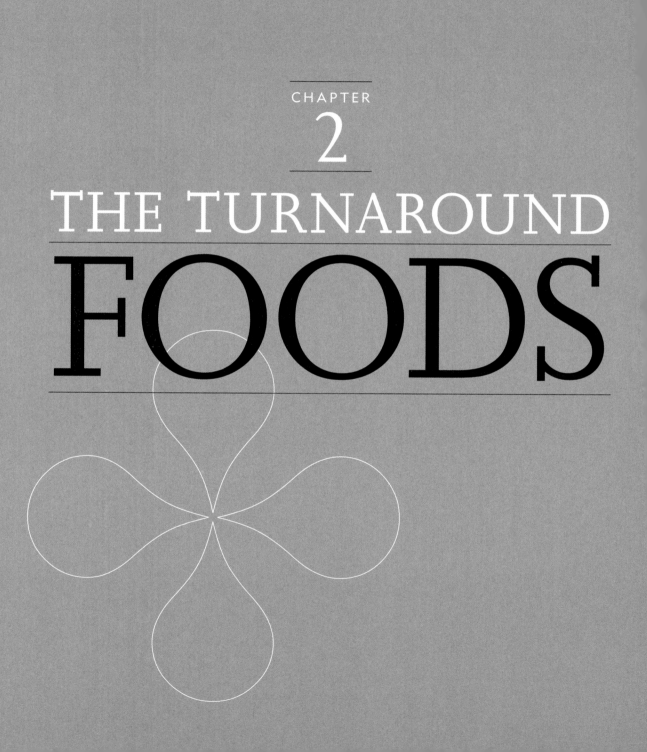

CHAPTER

2

THE TURNAROUND
FOODS

When you hear the word *diet*, does it make you want to run in the opposite direction? You're not alone. Many women have given up on shedding extra weight—frustrated with the time and effort put into fad diets that are impossible to follow for more than a few days. Don't run away just yet though, as this eating plan is different. It's a sustainable way of eating that is built on changing your habits. Even better, the plan is customizable, so you can mix and match foods to fit your needs. The end result? You're much more likely to stick to—and enjoy—this eating plan for life.

The recipes in this eating plan have been balanced to provide you with the maximum amount of energy and nutrients, while helping you to lose weight at the same time. Your goal on this diet is to eat about 1,600 calories a day, in the form of three healthy meals and two satisfying snacks. Your daily calories will be made up of carbs (about 45 percent), fat (about 25 percent), and protein (30 percent). *Note:* For men on this plan, the total calorie count is 2,000 (400 calories per meal and 400 calories per snack).

Following this kind of diet—one that's lower in calories, with moderate amounts of carbs and fat, and higher amounts of protein—can help you lose weight, particularly if you time when you eat.[1] And this type of eating plan won't leave you feeling fatigued. The meals and snacks have been created to keep your hunger in check and optimize your energy, since each one is nutritionally balanced. So you'll have all the fuel you need to make it through your day—and your workouts![2]

Specifically, on each day of this diet, you'll be choosing to eat the following Turnaround Food Choices:

- 4 servings of vegetables
- 2 servings of fruit
- 4 servings of grains/starchy vegetables
- 3 servings of dairy
- 3 servings of protein
- 3 servings of fat

"ALL MEANINGFUL AND LASTING CHANGE STARTS FIRST IN YOUR IMAGINATION AND THEN WORKS ITS WAY OUT."

—ALBERT EINSTEIN

For those of you who don't want to think about organizing your meals, or just need some time to get the hang of this plan, we lay out 2 full weeks of suggested menus. But we realize that not everyone will love all of the recommended recipes, so you're free to swap out a meal for one you find more appetizing. It's really that easy! If you'd rather create your own menus, you're free to mix and match options until you find a food combo that works for you. As long as your daily menu consists of three meals and two snacks that include the Turnaround Food Choices (see the chart starting on page 22), it fits into our eating plan.

The whole point of this diet is to enjoy what you're eating, so you'll actually *want* to continue eating this way after you've completed the 2 weeks. Food is not only fuel for everything we do—including the 2-Week Total Body Turnaround workouts—it's something we should enjoy, too!

Keep It Whole

Before getting into the specifics of what you'll be eating on this diet plan, I want to talk about what you *won't* be eating. The *2-Week Turnaround Diet Cookbook* is based on eating whole foods as often as possible. This means sticking to quality foods that are as close to their natural state as possible, while getting rid of options that are chock-full of preservatives, additives, processed sugars, chemicals, and general junk. Why? These processed and lower-quality foods can confuse our bodies and mess with our hormones, potentially resulting in extra body fat and illnesses such as heart disease and diabetes.

The first step to success on this diet plan is to eliminate all those diet-derailing junk-food temptations! How? Go through your cupboards, shelves, fridge, and freezer and throw out—don't just hide—foods such as ice cream, chips, candy, and cookies. The last thing you need while trying to establish new, healthy eating habits are junk foods that can entice you in a moment of weakness. If nothing else, at least get rid of your "trigger" foods—you know, the ones that can kick off binge or unhealthy eating. For me, my trigger food is candy, so I simply avoid it in the grocery store!

Now that your kitchen has been cleared, it's time to fill it with the whole foods that make up this eating plan. These are nutrient-dense foods that will keep your body running at its best and maximize your workouts. We're talking about foods such as fresh fruits and vegetables, whole grains, low-fat or fat-free dairy, healthy fats, lean meats, poultry, and fish. Having these foods on hand, plus other smart snacks, will help ensure that you stay on the healthy-eating track during the next 2 weeks. So eliminate unhealthy choices, and make a habit of feeding your body only the good stuff.

Breaking Down the Diet

Your kitchen is now free of unhealthful foods. Doesn't it feel liberating? Now we can shift gears and take a closer look at the healthy and nutrient-dense foods you will be eating during the next 2 weeks—and hopefully for a lifetime!

Eat a Rainbow: Fruits and Veggies

You'll be eating four servings of vegetables (see page 22) and two servings of fruit (see page 23) every day while on this plan. By now you've surely heard of all the amazing ways that fruits and veggies can boost your health. Not only do these superfoods contain essential vitamins, minerals, and fiber, but they are also low in calories. It doesn't stop there, though! Studies have shown that compared with people who consume only small amounts of fruits and vegetables in their diets, those who eat more generous amounts as part of a healthful diet are more likely to have a reduced risk of chronic diseases, including stroke and possibly other cardiovascular diseases, as well as certain cancers.[3]

Fruits and veggies also contain many other good-for-you compounds. For example, most fruits and veggies contain phytochemicals, chemicals that are produced by plants. More than 900 different phytochemicals, such as various carotenoids, flavonoids, phenolic compounds, and phytosterols, have been found in plant foods—and more are being discovered all the time. Research indicates that phytochemicals, when working with nutrients found in fruits and veggies, may help slow down the aging process and reduce the risk of many diseases, such as cancer, heart disease, stroke, high blood pressure, osteoporosis, urinary tract infections, and cataracts.[4]

Though the jury is still out on whether these health effects are due specifically to phytochemicals, you can't really go wrong by loading up on fruits and veggies.[5] When choosing which ones to eat, keep in mind that phytochemicals are usually related to plant pigments, so bright-colored fruits and veggies—think yellow, orange, red, green, blue, and purple—are excellent choices. Berries, grapes, carrots, broccoli, and tomatoes, for example, are packed with phytochemicals. You'll also find phytochemicals in grains, beans, nuts, and seeds

Many phytochemicals are also antioxidants. You've likely heard of these compounds, but what exactly are they? They are dietary substances, vitamins, and other nutrients that fight free radicals. Here's what happens: When our cells use oxygen, a process known as oxidation, they naturally produce unstable molecules called free radicals. These resulting free radicals

Linda Agnes
2-WEEK RESULTS:

**12 pounds,
16 inches lost**

DESPERATE FOR a change, Linda signed up to take the 2-week challenge. The first 2 days, she says, were the hardest. "I just started to cry when I realized how emotionally dependent I had become on food." But, she reports, something happened on Day 3: "My brain suddenly cleared. After 3 days of working out and eating healthfully, it felt like I woke up from some kind of coma and was starting anew." Linda intends to follow the program for the rest of her life. "This has ignited a positive change in my life, both physically and mentally. I know exactly what I need to do now to get results, and I know I will get there."

can roam around in our bodies, starting a chain reaction that damages cells, and they may play a role in heart disease, cancer, and other diseases.[6] These free radicals can also be produced in small amounts when you do aerobic exercise, such as jogging or running.[7] You don't want to stop exercising, though, since you know aerobic exercise has many health benefits and really energizes you. So how can you combat free radicals?

A diet rich in antioxidants, like those found in fruits and vegetables, can help counteract this damage. How? Antioxidants slow down or prevent oxidation because they can stabilize free radicals before the substances react and cause harm. The most well-known antioxidants include such nutrients as beta-carotene, vitamin A (found in liver, dairy, and fish), vitamin C (found in bell peppers and citrus fruits), vitamin E (found in oils, fortified cereals, seeds, and nuts), and the mineral selenium (found in meats, tuna, and plant foods). Lots of fruits and veggies contain antioxidants, including berries (blueberries, blackberries, raspberries, strawberries, and cranberries are among the top sources of antioxidants), many apple varieties (eat them with the peel), avocados, cherries, artichokes, spinach, and broccoli—again, think rainbow![8] Antioxidants are also found in nuts, grains, and some meats, poultry, and fish.

To get the full spectrum of nutrients and other beneficial compounds found in fruits and veggies, our eating plan suggests you aim for at least three different colors of veggies each day and two different colors of fruits. So mix it up—the more colorful the better! When buying fruits and veggies, try to go for the freshest produce available, which often means eating foods that are in season. Farmers markets and food cooperatives are a great place to get fresh and seasonal fruits and veggies. And don't hesitate to ask someone at your local grocery store for help in selecting the freshest stuff.

Go for Complex Carbs: Starchy Veggies and Grains

You'll be eating four servings of grains or starchy vegetables (see page 22)—both of which are complex carbohydrates—every day on this eating plan. We recommend that you choose three whole grain foods (such as whole wheat bread and pasta, and brown rice) and one starchy veggie (these are veggies with a lot of substance that will fill you up fast, such as beans, plantains, and sweet potatoes).

These starchy, complex carbs are an essential part of your diet, allowing for proper organ function and providing the fuel needed to maximize your workouts. In fact, carbs are the easiest source of fuel for our bodies to use. Here's how they work: Carbs are broken down in our bodies into simple sugars that enter the bloodstream and are converted into glucose. This glucose is your body's first choice for fuel, and whatever isn't used up immediately is stored as glycogen in the liver and muscles. Your muscles tap into your glycogen reserves when they need energy. When eaten in moderation, carbs can help keep you fired up all day long. For this reason, you'll be getting about 45 percent of your daily calories from carbs in our plan—enough to maintain energy levels for your workouts.

Not all carbs are the same, however. In general, the longer a carbohydrate takes to break down in our bodies, the healthier it is. This is what the "good" carbs versus "bad" carbs debate centers around. Nutritionists use a scale called the glycemic index (GI) to measure how quickly a food will release sugars into the bloodstream. The higher the GI number, the faster the food breaks down and enters your bloodstream. Simple carbs, such as white bread, white rice, white potatoes, cookies, and sugary sodas, are digested quickly, so they cause a spike in blood-sugar levels. Complex carbs, on the other hand, such as whole grains, beans, veggies, and oats, take longer for the body to break down and digest, keeping blood-sugar levels more stable. This GI difference can add or subtract inches from your waistline. Often, the body can't break down a high-GI food fast enough, so the carbs get stored as fat and the metabolism slows down. The resulting high blood-sugar levels from these carbs also cause increased levels of the hormone insulin, which can lead to weight gain because of increased hunger.[9] But with a low-GI food, your body has enough time to break down the carbohydrates without having them stored as fat. The slower release of sugars into the bloodstream also has less of an impact on insulin levels.

So the trick with carbs is to pick the right type, as it can make all the difference in your health and workout plan. That's why we focus on whole grains rather than refined grains. All grains actually start out whole, but when refined, the bran and germ—which contain important nutrients— are removed. Whole grains, on the other hand, contain the entire grain kernel—the bran, germ, and endosperm. While all types of grains contain various vitamins and minerals and are naturally low in fat, whole grains are a better source of fiber and other important nutrients, such as selenium, potassium, and magnesium.[10] These whole grains include whole wheat bread and pasta, brown or wild rice, oatmeal, and grains like quinoa or bulgur. If you want to branch out, you can also try barley, buckwheat, corn on the cob, millet, amaranth, and wheat berries.

Whole grains not only taste delicious, they also contain antioxidants and have a host of health benefits. A diet high in whole grains has been linked to a lower risk of cardiovascular disease, type 2 diabetes, and cancer.[11] And because whole grains are full of fiber, they will help keep your digestive system in check, boost your health by lowering "bad" LDL cholesterol levels, and allow you to feel full and satisfied for longer. The *2-Week Turnaround Diet Cookbook* allows you to take advantage of fiber's benefits by providing about 25 grams a day.

These good-for-you grains can also have a favorable effect on your weight. Emerging evidence suggests that eating whole grains may contribute to achieving and maintaining a healthy weight.[12] One 12-year study found that women who consistently consumed more whole grains weighed less than women who consumed fewer whole grains; those who ate the most fiber had a lower risk of major weight gain.[13] Another study, this one in men, showed that eating whole grains and bran might reduce long-term weight gain.[14]

You'll notice on page 22 that starchy vegetables, like sweet potatoes, plantains, corn, peas, and beans, are listed with the grains. These veggies are high in carbohydrates (a serving has about as many carbs as a slice of bread). They're still extremely good for you, and you can absolutely eat them in this plan, but just remember to count them as a grain serving.

Do It Right: Dairy

You'll consume three servings of dairy or dairy substitutes (see page 23) a day on this plan: one at breakfast and two as snacks. Dairy products are among the best sources of calcium, a mineral that is important for healthy bones and teeth, as well as for the proper functioning of your heart, muscles, and nerves. Your body can't produce calcium, so it must be absorbed through the foods you eat.[15] Since getting enough calcium is vital to maximizing bone health, the mineral plays a crucial role in preventing the bone disease osteoporosis, which leads to an increased risk of bone fractures. Here's the deal: Our bones are constantly being built up and broken down. By around the age of 20, the average woman has acquired the greatest amount of bone she will ever have, a point called the peak bone mass.[16] In fact, about 85 to 90 percent of adult bone mass is acquired by age 18 in girls and age 20 in boys.[17] And although the bone tissue can keep growing until around 30, after this point, you slowly start to lose more bone than you can build.

Getting enough calcium and being physically active during these critical years allows you to build strong bones and maximize your bone mass before this natural decline starts. Vitamin D—which milk is fortified with—also plays an important role in healthy bone development because it helps in the absorption of calcium. Consuming enough of these nutrients, which is easy if you eat our suggested dairy servings, may reduce the risk of osteoporosis later in life.[18] An estimated 8 million women and 2 million men have osteoporosis, with an additional 34 million at risk.[19]

Postmenopausal women are especially at risk, because estrogen levels, which are important in maintaining bone health, start to decline at menopause. Dairy doesn't just build strong bones and teeth; it may also lower the risk of developing high blood pressure and heart disease.[20] But to truly reap dairy's health benefits, you want to stick with low-fat and fat-free options, as this will cut the fat from your diet and keep your calories in check. Smart dairy options include fat-free milk, yogurt, cottage cheese, ricotta cheese, and other part-skim or reduced-fat cheeses. Full-fat dairy items are also high in saturated fat, which can raise blood cholesterol and lead to heart disease. The low-fat and fat-free dairy options taste just as delicious, while keeping your heart healthy.

Need another reason to love calcium? Here's one: Studies have shown it may also play an important role in weight loss. One study found that people who followed a diet that included 800 milligrams of calcium supplements per day lost significantly more weight than those who had only about half that amount of calcium in their diets; those who got their calcium from dairy products (three servings a day, or about 1,200 to 1,300 milligrams of calcium) lost even more weight.[21]

Other research has seemed to show that when exercising adults on a slightly reduced-calorie diet consumed three to four servings of dairy daily (versus one serving), their metabolism changed so that they burned more fat.[22] While more recent studies dispute these claims, leaving the dairy and weight-loss connection up in the air, it shouldn't hurt your waistline to add dairy to your diet, as long as you eat it in moderation and stick with low-fat options.[23]

On this plan, protein and dairy are grouped separately. But dairy foods are also great sources of high-quality protein, providing all of the essential amino acids you need to build and repair your muscles. As we explain in "Timing Is Everything" on page 3, for a pre- or post-workout snack (when

DAIRY FREE? NO PROBLEM!

IF DAIRY DOESN'T AGREE with you, no worries. There are lots of nondairy options that are chock-full of calcium, such as dark green leafy vegetables (try bok choy, broccoli, or kale) and nuts (try almonds). Many foods are also fortified with calcium, including orange juice, cereal, soy beverages, and tofu products.[24] (Tofu prepared with calcium sulfate contains more calcium than tofu made with nigari. Read the ingredients list.) Check out the vegan section at your supermarket—there's nondairy cheese, soy and coconut milk yogurt, and even soy ice cream! Just remember that plant-based foods generally have less bioavailability, which means it's a little harder for your body to absorb the calcium from these sources.

you'll want to include protein), any of the dairy-containing savory snacks on this plan are perfect.

Power Up: Protein

You'll eat three servings of lean protein (see page 24) on this meal plan, one at each meal. We encourage you to choose fish two or three times a week as your protein option, as well as a vegetarian source (you can try tofu, veggie burgers, or tempeh, for example) at least twice a week. Keep in mind that while other foods in this diet plan provide protein—such as dairy products and beans—these three servings of lean protein are in addition to the other sources of protein. Protein is essential for building and repairing muscles.

The Institute of Medicine (a nonprofit organization that works to provide unbiased, authoritative advice to the public and to government decision makers) recommends that adults get a minimum of 0.8 gram of protein daily for every kilogram of body weight—that's about 8 grams of protein for every 20 pounds of weight.[25] When we eat protein, it's broken down by our bodies into molecules called amino acids. There are about 20 amino acids in total, and these are the building blocks of protein. While fats and carbs can be stored, our bodies can't hold on to amino acids. This means you need a fresh supply of amino acids every day to keep your body working at its full potential. About half of these amino acids can't be made by our bodies, so they have to come from our diet— these are known as the essential amino acids. By eating a variety of protein sources, such as those found in our meal plan, you should be able to get all the amino acids you need.

The protein in your meals and snacks also slightly boosts your metabolism. Here's why: Protein has the same number of calories per gram as carbs (4 calories per gram) and less than half that of fat (which has 9 calories per gram). But since your body has to break down each gram of protein into its individual amino acids, it takes more energy and more time to digest. It actually takes our bodies about three times more energy to digest protein than to digest carbs or fat. This slower digestion process not only benefits your metabolism, it also helps keep you feeling full for longer and won't raise your blood-sugar levels as quickly as high-GI carbs, like white rice and white potatoes.

Protein also plays an important role when you're working out. While carbs are the fuel for your workouts, protein provides the muscle-building power. The amino acids from protein are used primarily for building and repairing muscles, though your body can break down muscle tissue to provide energy in an emergency. Strength training is an essential part of the

2-Week Total Body Turnaround exercise program, and you'll be working your muscles especially hard on 12 of the plan's 14 days. So you must provide your muscles with all the necessary power to get strong and sculpted during these sessions. Most active women should be eating a diet of at least 15 to 30 percent protein. On our 1,600-calorie diet program, 30 percent of your calories will come from protein. If you combine a protein-rich diet with the exercises, you'll start to see your muscles grow!

If you want to further maximize the results of our exercise program, choose one of the protein-rich meals or snacks during the hour after you work out. This period immediately after exercise, known as the glycogen window, is when the muscles are better able to absorb glucose and store it as glycogen. As you know, dairy foods are great sources of protein. When selecting your post-workout snack, choose any of the savory snacks (to keep your blood sugar consistent and prevent energy crashes) on this plan that contain dairy. Choose snacks with the note, "This recipe makes a good pre/post workout snack."

Protein-rich dishes are also a good source of iron, which provides energy and is used by red blood cells to transport oxygen throughout the body. When a person doesn't get enough iron, they can feel lazy and tired. This is the case for many premenopausal women, since they can lose a lot of iron if they have heavy periods. Some seafoods and lean meats are good sources of iron, including lean beef, turkey, lamb, chicken, clams, and oysters. If you're not a meat eater, you can try soy products, dark leafy greens such as spinach and kale, fortified whole grain cereals, lentils, and beans. To maximize your iron absorption, be sure to eat these iron-rich foods with foods that are high in vitamin C (like oranges or orange juice). Why? Vitamin C helps in iron absorption.

These benefits of eating protein are not a green light for you to go overboard, however. If you eat too much protein, as with all foods, it will be stored as fat. You also have to be careful because protein-rich foods are often high in fat, especially artery-clogging saturated fat. Eating too much red meat has been associated with health risks such as increased "bad" LDL cholesterol and total cholesterol, heart attack and stroke, and certain cancers, and red meat is a source of several cancer-causing compounds.[26] So this eating plan gives you enough protein to reap the nutrient's benefits without going overboard.

To make the most of your protein servings in this diet, stick to lean meats, such as sirloin or pork tenderloin, as well as chicken breast or turkey. Seafood is also a great option, including tuna, salmon, or shrimp. If you don't eat meat, you can still load up on protein. Go for smart veggie options such as tofu and other soy products, beans, nuts, and eggs.

REAL 2-WEEK TURNAROUND SUCCESS STORY

Michelle Knapek
2-WEEK RESULTS:
**6 pounds,
11¾ inches lost**

WHEN THE scale remained stuck despite a few attempts at weight loss, Michelle knew she had to change something. Adding more vegetables to her diet and making healthier meal choices helped her lose 6 pounds and 11¾ inches, including a remarkable 3 inches from her waist in just 2 weeks. A few days into the plan, she began to see a difference. "The first thing I noticed was the puffiness in my face and body went down. Then I found I was sleeping better. And the greatest change was that it nearly completely alleviated all of those miserable menopausal symptoms."

Find the Flavor: Fat

You'll be eating three servings of healthy fats a day on this plan, one at each meal. We recommend that you choose plant-based fats over meat-based ones as often as possible, and aim for variety.

Fats do not make you fat. In fact, everyone needs to eat some fat to fully absorb certain vitamins, and fats provide you with lots of energy. While carbs are our bodies' main source of fuel (including for your workouts), fats are the backup fuel source. Fats are broken down by our bodies into fatty acids, which can be converted into energy, but the process takes longer than it does with carbs. This makes fatty acids a better energy source for lower-intensity exercise, such as walking. When fatty acids aren't used as energy, they are stored as, well, fat. Unfortunately, glycogen—the stored form of glucose found in the muscles—can only be stored in relatively small amounts, but there's no limit to how much fat our bodies can amass. Clearly this isn't good news, especially for women, as we often see this fat end up on our hips, butt, and thighs. Since fats are calorically dense (remember, 1 gram of fat has 9 calories, compared to only 4 calories per gram in carbs and protein), you need to be extra careful about how much you eat—the calories can add up fast! So the fat content in this eating plan, about 25 percent of your daily calories, is high enough to keep you satisfied, curb cravings, and maximize the flavor in your food, but low enough to see real results from your workouts.

As with carbs, though, all fats are not created equal and the type you eat will make all the difference in your health—and your waistline. After years of warning us about the dangers of fat, researchers now realize that there are actually "good" fats. These good guys are called unsaturated fats, and they've been shown to boost our health in many ways, including improving cholesterol levels, reducing inflammation, lowering the risk of certain cancers, and maintaining brain health.

There are two types of unsaturated fats: monounsaturated and polyunsaturated. Yes, they're both a mouthful! You can find monounsaturated fats (we call them MUFAs) in foods such as avocados and peanut butter; canola, olive, and peanut oils; pistachios, almonds, and other nuts; and various seeds. Last but not least, you can even find MUFAs in—drumroll, please—dark chocolate! It's true. These MUFAs have wide-ranging potential health benefits, including protecting your heart.

Polyunsaturated fats, meanwhile, aren't too shabby themselves in the health department. These fats are found in foods such as vegetable oils (like soybean, sunflower, and corn oils), as well as walnuts, flaxseed, and some fish. One polyunsaturated fat in particular has reached superstar status—omega-3 fatty acid. It's hard to miss the news about omega-3s these days, as they've been associated with everything from reducing arthritis and inflammation to improving heart health. Omega-3s are found in high amounts in fatty, cold-water fish such as salmon, mackerel, and herring.

For all these reasons, this eating plan includes moderate amounts of these healthy, good fats. What it doesn't include, though, are unhealthy fats. Who are these bad guys? Saturated and trans fats. Both types of fat can harm your health and are responsible for fat's continued bad reputation. You can find saturated fats mostly in animal products, such as meat and whole-milk dairy products (cheese, milk, butter, cream, and even premium ice cream), as well as a few plant-based foods like coconut oil, palm oil, and cocoa butter. These fats can be harmful to your heart, as they are known to boost "bad" LDL cholesterol levels and have been linked to coronary heart disease.[27]

If you think saturated fats are bad, though, be prepared for trans fatty acids, aka trans fats. These bad boys are created when liquid oils are converted into solid fats. This is done by heating vegetable oils in the presence of hydrogen, a process known as hydrogenation. Why in the world would you do this to a fat? It creates a partially hydrogenated oil (look for the words *partially hydrogenated* on a food label to identify trans fats), which is a more stable fat that can allow food to stay fresh for longer. While this is great news for food manufacturers who don't want their foods to spoil quickly, it's not such good news for you. These trans fats can increase "bad" LDL cholesterol, while decreasing "good" HDL cholesterol—and both scenarios are risk factors for heart disease.[28]

You'll find trans fats most often in fried foods and commercial baked goods such as cookies, crackers, and pies. In 2006, food manufacturers were required to list them on the Nutrition Facts label, and in response, many companies are scrambling to get rid of these fats. Be aware, though, that even foods touted as "trans fat free" on their labels can have up to 0.5 gram of trans-fats, which will add up over time.

Drink It Up: Water

Last, but certainly not least, don't forget water! On this plan you'll be drinking lots of this thirst-quenching stuff—at least one glass with each of your meals and snacks, for a total of 2 liters a day. Don't wait until you're thirsty to drink, as you'll need extra water to keep up with your daily physical activity. So get in the habit of carrying a bottle of water around, and drink it regularly throughout the day, particularly when you're eating and working out. The best part? It's calorie free!

It's vital to consume enough water every day because you'll find this good stuff in every cell, tissue, and organ in your body. Water helps keep you feeling energized, helps you feel fuller, improves your workouts, and may even help you eat less. One study found that people who drank water before meals ate about 75 fewer calories at each meal. If you subtract 75 calories from one meal every day for a year, you could lose almost 8 pounds—all this just by reaching for your water glass![29] And a German study showed that after drinking 17 ounces of water (just a little more than a regular-size water bottle), volunteers' metabolisms increased by an average of 30 percent.[30]

Drinking water while working out will help prevent dehydration. Your body produces heat when you're physically active, which exits your body in the form of sweat. If you don't replace these fluids, your heart rate will go up, as well as your body temperature. This not only can compromise your workout, but it also puts you at risk of becoming dehydrated. So it's essential to load up on water while exercising.[31]

If water is too plain for you, fear not. You can make it tastier by drinking flavored water. Not the artificial, store-bought kind—instead, create your own simple version by adding healthy options such as slices of cucumber, orange, lemon, lime, grapefruit, or even mint leaves to a jug of water. Let your concoction sit for a while so the flavors infuse, and then enjoy! It's an easy way to add a little flavor.

Water is your best bet for staying adequately hydrated over the next 2 weeks. Despite all the hype, there's no need for energy drinks during your workouts, particularly since many of these beverages contain a lot of caffeine and will only lead to quick, short-lived energy bursts. The only time when drinking water alone may not be enough is if you're working out for more than an hour a day or exercising in extremely hot conditions. In those cases, a sports drink may be in order. Even then, though, stay away from typical energy drinks and go for a sports beverage like Gatorade instead. These types of drinks can provide the necessary carbs to give you that extra boost, as well as electrolytes to replace minerals lost through sweat. But unlike water, these drinks aren't calorie free—even 8 ounces of Gatorade has 50 calories. Only water can provide the hydration without the calories.

Take Control

Portion control is everything when it comes to making good food choices. Almonds are among the healthiest foods out there, but if you eat the entire tin, you'll consume about 1,500 calories or more! Many of our test panelists found that keeping a set of measuring cups on the counter helped them to figure out the right amount that they should be eating with each meal or snack. Here are some good guidelines to keep in mind:

- Your fist = a medium portion of fruit or 1 cup of rice or pasta
- Your thumb = a 1-ounce serving of cheese
- The tip of your thumb = 1 teaspoon of butter or oil
- A deck of cards = a 3-ounce serving of meat, poultry, or fish
- One cupped handful = 1 serving of cereal, pretzels, or chips

SODIUM SAVVY

THE USDA DIETARY GUIDELINES recommend a maximum of 2,300 milligrams of sodium per day—that's about 1 teaspoon of salt. Currently, the average sodium intake is about 4,000 milligrams a day, nearly twice the recommended level.

So what's the problem with too much salt? A large study called DASH (Dietary Approaches to Stop Hypertension) from the National Heart, Lung, and Blood Institute found that when people cut their sodium levels, they also reduced high blood pressure. The biggest changes came when people consumed just 1,500 milligrams of sodium a day. Following a low-sodium diet (along with eating plenty of fruits, vegetables, and whole grains) was estimated to reduce heart disease by 15 percent and stroke by 27 percent.

Surprisingly, the saltshaker isn't the main culprit for the high amount of sodium in the American diet. Restaurant meals and processed foods (like lunchmeats, canned soups, frozen meals, condiments, shelf-stable meals, crackers, and instant cereals) are the real sodium offenders.

You can greatly lower your sodium consumption simply by eating whole foods. And you'll limit your total sodium intake if you limit the frequency with which you eat away from home. You'll see in our suggested menus, by the way, that we recommend no more than 600 to 650 milligrams of sodium in each meal (and no more than 150 to 200 milligrams of sodium in each snack) to stay under the 2,300-milligram-a-day level. However, you'll also see that there are a few meals that go beyond that range. As usual, you can always make exceptions to any nutrition rule as long as you keep things balanced overall, so just be sure the other meals you select in that day are a little lower in sodium. In addition, because you'll be sweating a lot during this 2-week program, a little extra sodium during this time isn't likely to be a problem!

TURNAROUND FOOD CHOICES

Here are the building blocks for your 2-Week Turnaround Diet.

Vegetables

Number of servings per day: 4; 2 at lunch, 2 at dinner; aim for at least 3 different colors each day

Fresh, 1 serving equals 1 cup raw or ½ cup cooked:
- Artichokes
- Arugula
- Asparagus
- Bok choy
- Broccoli
- Broccoli rabe
- Brussels sprouts
- Cabbage
- Carrots
- Cauliflower
- Celery
- Chard
- Coleslaw mix
- Collard greens
- Cucumbers
- Eggplant
- Green beans
- Jicama
- Kale
- Leeks
- Lettuce, all types
- Mushrooms
- Okra
- Onions
- Peppers
- Radicchio
- Radishes
- Shallots
- Spaghetti squash
- Spinach
- Summer squash
- Tomatillos
- Tomatoes
- Watercress
- Zucchini

Canned or jarred, 1 serving equals ½ cup:
- Artichoke hearts, in water
- Roasted red peppers, in water
- Salsa
- Tomatoes, stewed or diced
- Tomato sauce

Frozen, 1 serving equals 1 cup before cooking:
- Asparagus
- Broccoli
- Brussels sprouts
- Carrots
- Cauliflower
- Green beans
- Kale
- Mushrooms
- Okra
- Spinach
- Sugar snap peas
- Yellow wax beans

Grains/Starchy Vegetables

Number of servings per day: 4; 2 at breakfast, 1 at lunch, 1 at dinner; aim for 3 whole grain servings and 1 starchy veggie daily

Starchy vegetables, 1 serving equals ½ cup cooked:
- Beans, all varieties (black, kidney, lima, pinto, refried, etc.)
- Beets
- Corn
- Fava beans
- Lentils
- Parsnips
- Peas
- Plantains
- Potatoes, red
- Potatoes, sweet
- Winter squashes (butternut, acorn, etc.)

Breads, 1 serving equals:
- Bread, whole grain, 1 slice
- English muffin, whole grain, 1 half
- Pita, 100% oat bran or whole wheat, 1 half
- Tortillas, corn, 2
- Wrap, 100% whole grain, 1 half

Frozen grains or starchy veggies, 1 serving equals:
- Corn, white or yellow, ½ cup heated
- Green peas, ½ cup heated
- Lima beans, ½ cup heated
- Pancakes, whole grain, 1
- Waffles, whole grain, 1

Grains, 1 serving equals:
- Bulgur, ½ cup cooked
- Cereal, whole grain, ½ cup dry
- Couscous, ½ cup cooked
- Crackers, whole grain, ½ cup
- Cream of wheat, ½ cup cooked
- Farro, ½ cup cooked
- Oatmeal, ½ cup cooked

- Pasta, whole wheat, ½ cup cooked
- Popcorn, light microwave (no trans fat), 3 cups popped
- Quinoa, ½ cup cooked
- Rice, brown or wild, ½ cup cooked

Fruits

Number of servings per day: 2; 1 at breakfast, 1 as a snack; aim for 2 different colors each day

**Fresh, 1 serving
equals 1 cup or
1 medium piece
the size of
your fist:**

- Apples, all varieties
- Apricots
- Bananas, small
- Blackberries
- Blueberries
- Cantaloupe
- Cherries
- Clementines
- Dates
- Figs
- Grapefruit
- Grapes
- Guavas
- Honeydew melon
- Kiwifruit
- Mangoes
- Nectarines
- Oranges
- Papayas
- Passion fruit
- Peaches
- Pears
- Pineapple
- Plums
- Pomegranates
- Raspberries
- Star fruit
- Strawberries
- Tangerines
- Watermelon

**Frozen, 1 serving
equals 1 cup in
frozen state:**

- Any unsweetened
  variety, including:
- Blackberries
- Blueberries
- Cherries
- Mangoes
- Peaches
- Pineapple
- Raspberries
- Strawberries

**Canned, 1 serving
equals ½ cup:**

- Any unsweetened
  variety, in natural
  juice:
- Applesauce,
  natural
- Apricots
- Fruit juice, 100%
- Mandarin oranges
- Mixed fruit
- Peaches
- Pears
- Pineapple
- Plums

**Dried, 1 serving
equals ½ cup,
unsweetened:**

- Apples
- Apricots
- Bananas
- Blueberries
- Cherries
- Dates
- Figs
- Mangoes
- Peaches
- Pears
- Pineapple
- Plums
- Raisins, regular or
  golden

Dairy or Dairy Substitutes

Number of servings per day: 3; 1 at breakfast, 2 as snacks; use only fat-free milk, yogurt, cottage cheese, and ricotta cheese, and reduced-fat cheeses

**Reduced-fat
crumbled or
shredded cheese—
1 serving equals
¼ cup:**

- Blue
- Cheddar
- Colby
- Feta
- Fontina
- Gorgonzola
- Gruyère
- Jack
- Mozzarella
- Parmesan
- Romano
- Vegan cheese
  substitutes

**Reduced-fat sliced
cheese, 1 serving
equals 1 slice,
about the size of a
coaster:**

- American
- Cheddar
- Gouda
- Jack
- Mozzarella
- Provolone
- Swiss
- Vegan cheese
  substitutes

**Others, 1 serving
equals:**

- Cottage cheese,
  nonfat, ½ cup
- Milk, fat-free, 1 cup
- Ricotta, nonfat,
  ½ cup
- Soy, rice, or
  almond milk, 1 cup
  (check to make
  sure it's fortified
  with calcium)
- String cheese,
  1 string
- Yogurt, Greek or
  regular, fat-free,
  low-fat, or soy,
  1 cup

[CONTINUED]

TURNAROUND FOOD CHOICES [CONTINUED]

Protein

Number of servings per day: 3; 1 at breakfast, lunch, and dinner; choose fish 2 or 3 times a week and a vegetarian source (tofu, veggie burgers) at least twice a week

Unless otherwise stated, 1 serving equals 3 ounces or 1 piece about the size of a cassette tape or a deck of cards, cooked or prepared:

- Beef, ground, 98% lean or leaner
- Beef tenderloin
- Canadian bacon
- Chicken breast

- Chicken sausage, low-fat
- Chicken thighs, skinless
- Clams, fresh, or minced, canned
- Crab, fresh
- Duck breast, skinless
- Egg whites, 1 cup liquid or whites from 5 eggs

- Fish, fresh (halibut, cod, snapper, flounder, etc.)
- Ham, deli meat, lean
- Lobster, fresh
- Mussels, fresh
- Oysters, fresh
- Pork tenderloin
- Roast beef, deli meat, lean
- Salmon, wild, fresh or canned

- Shrimp, frozen or canned
- Sirloin, trimmed
- Soy-based vegetarian products (tofu, veggie burgers, dogs, patties, bacon, etc.)
- Tuna, chunk light, canned in water
- Turkey, deli meat

- Turkey, ground, leanest possible
- Turkey bacon
- Turkey breast
- Turkey sausage, low-fat

Fat

Number of servings per day: 3; 1 at breakfast, lunch, and dinner; choose plant-based fats as often as possible and aim for variety

1 serving equals:

- Avocado, 1/5 of medium size
- Cream cheese, light or reduced fat, 2 Tbsp

- Mayonnaise, light or reduced fat, 2 Tbsp
- Nut butters, including peanut, cashew, almond, soy, or walnut butter, 2 Tbsp

- Nuts or seeds, chopped or sliced, including walnuts, almonds, pecans, peanuts, cashews, pistachios, pine nuts, sunflower seeds, pumpkin seeds, 2 Tbsp

- Oil-based salad dressings, 2 Tbsp
- Olives, 10 medium, black or green
- Pesto, 1 Tbsp

- Vegetable oils, including olive, canola, sunflower, peanut, sesame, 1 Tbsp

Beverages—Water

Number of servings per day: 2 liters; drink with each meal; don't rely on thirst to guide your intake—carry a water bottle or pour a glass with each of your 3 meals and 2 snacks

In addition to the 2 liters of water, you can have the following noncaloric beverages:

- Coffee, black
- Seltzer or sparkling water
- Tea, black

- Tea, green
- Tea, herbal

Note: Coffee and black and green tea contain caffeine and are mild diuretics (they cause the body to lose water), so they should be limited to around 2 cups per day.

Eating Out Know-How

From all-American diners to the most international cuisines, there's always a good eating-out choice available for you. The tips below will help you make waistline-friendly choices.

● **GET INFORMED.** Many restaurants post their entire menu plus nutrition information online, making it easy to make an informed choice.

● **GET A CLUE.** The description on the menu can tell you a lot about how a food is prepared. Words like *fried, battered, crispy, au gratin, scalloped,* and *creamed* usually mean big-time calories, plus trans or artery-clogging saturated fat. Instead, look for healthy key words like *grilled, blackened, baked, broiled* (but not in butter!), or *dry roasted.*

● **AVOID UNNECESSARY TEMPTATIONS.** If the tortilla chips or bread basket that is automatically brought to your table sabotages your best intentions before the meal officially starts, simply ask your server to keep it in the kitchen.

● **BE THE BOSS.** Want the grilled chicken club, but don't need the bacon, cheese, and mayo, as well as the accompanying fries? Order your meal "your way" by asking the server to hold off on the things you don't want, or inquire about substitutions. Almost all restaurants will be more than happy to accommodate your requests.

● **SPLIT IT OR SAVE IT.** Many restaurant meals are humongous. If you notice the meal is bigger than you need (and it probably is), ask your server to bring you a take-out container to divide your meal before you dig in. You'll have another meal for tomorrow! Better yet, split your meal with a dining companion.

● **GO SMALL.** Aim to choose the smallest portions when you can: a petite-cut steak, a small ice cream cone, a half of a sandwich. Diminutive meal portions can be supplemented with healthy extras like veggies, fruit, and broth-based soups, while small portions of desserts like ice cream can give you the flavor you crave without blowing your diet.

● **PUT IT ON THE SIDE.** Be sure you ask for sauces and dressings on the side, instead of having them added to your meal in the kitchen. You can control the amount you use, and enjoy the natural flavor of the foods without having them drowned in extra fat and calories.

PUTTING IT INTO
PRACTICE

d o you feel like a healthy eating expert yet? You should! You now have the lowdown on all of the types of nutrient-dense foods, and you're well on your way to learning how to create healthy habits for life. Over the next 14 days you'll be forced to look closely at your food-related behaviors, and then be challenged to make them better. Whether you're a healthy eating novice or a smart food guru, the 2-Week Turnaround Diet Cookbook will encourage healthier habits by providing food basics, tips, tricks, and an abundance of recipes. You'll start to feel your energy soar, your fitness levels improve, and your confidence rise. Are you ready?

Before we jump into the plan, let's look at some things you can do before you start the diet to make the next 2 weeks even easier and more successful. First things first, make sure you pick a good time in your life to start this diet. I know what you're thinking: Is there ever a good time to change the way you eat? But some times are actually better than others. This is an eating plan you can follow long after the 2 weeks are done, so you want to start off on the right foot. Having a good experience now may be all the motivation you need to continue with the plan, be it for another week or many more years. Remember, this diet—even when tweaked to make it better fit into your lifestyle—is a safe way to lose pounds in the long run, so take advantage of it for as long as possible.

What you want to do is kick off the eating plan at a time when you have 2 weeks to commit to it. This doesn't mean you must completely clear your schedule, but don't embark on the diet if you have upcoming events that will completely shake up your schedule—like a vacation or a demanding houseguest. Before you start to worry, though, rest assured that this plan won't take up all of your free time. But you do want to be able to invest some time in it, as it will help lay the foundation for healthy eating habits. In other words, make this plan the priority, even if only for 14 days! You'll be amazed at the habits that stick around long after you're done.

Let's look at other helpful things to do before you start the 2-week plan.

"THE SECRET OF SUCCESS IS CONSTANCY TO PURPOSE."

—BENJAMIN DISRAELI

Smart Shopping: Navigating the Aisles

Now that you've figured out the best moment to jump-start your new diet regimen, it's time to go shopping! Healthy eating begins with healthy grocery shopping, and what you put into your cart week after week can make all the difference in your health—and your waistline. Is your cart full of fruits, vegetables, and other whole foods that we recommend in this diet? Or is it overloaded with sugary products, unhealthy snacks, and processed foods? The trick to sticking with this eating plan is to ensure that those unhealthy foods don't even make it into your kitchen. Who needs the temptation? It's really important to head down the healthy eating path right from the start, and this begins in the grocery store.

Throughout this eating plan you'll be eating delicious recipes that are clearly laid out for you. In theory, it should be as simple as buying what's on the ingredients list, but I'm the first to admit that it can be intimidating to navigate those grocery store aisles. It's easy to get lost among the multitude of food options out there, not to mention the undecipherable food labels and abundance of health claims promising to change your life for the better. Then, of course, there are the enticing free samples and the sugary temptations waiting for you at the checkout counter. Put these factors together, and they can really make a dent in your wallet and lead to unwelcome pounds around your waist.

Luckily, there are little tricks you can use when you're food shopping to maximize your health and minimize your mishaps at the grocery store. To help you conquer the supermarket, try these tips:

- **MAKE A LIST:** Before you even set foot in the store, create a shopping list. Why? Because something as simple as a carefully crafted list of ingredients, especially if it's for a week's worth of meals, can make a big difference in your budget *and* your midsection. We've made it easy for you by doing the meal planning; now your task is to stick to the list. Don't get sidetracked by those unhealthy foods. Remember to double-check that you don't already have some of the ingredients in your pantry, fridge, or freezer before heading to the store. There's no reason to waste money!

- **FOLLOW THE HEALTHY PATH:** Believe it or not, the route you take in a grocery store can influence what you put in your shopping cart. Stick to the perimeter of the store as much as possible, since the outer aisles often contain the healthiest foods, such as fruits, veggies, dairy products, meat, and fish. You'll also find fewer products with confusing health claims in these aisles, since most fresh foods don't have labels. Once your cart is mostly full of foods from these aisles (say around three-quarters full), you can move to the inner aisles. Here you find the packaged and processed foods, often loaded with additives and artificial stuff. Stay away from these foods as much as possible, and focus on the healthier items found here instead, including canned beans, frozen fruits and veggies, whole grain products, and sauces. And don't just grab foods you see at eye level—scan the upper and lower shelves as well. Some manufacturers pay big money to get their newest products on the center shelves, but that doesn't mean they're the healthiest.

● **DON'T GO HUNGRY:** You've heard it before and we'll say it again: Don't go grocery shopping on an empty stomach. When you head to the store hungry, you're much more likely to load up on junk foods, which can be detrimental not only to your health, but also to your wallet. Suddenly every pie, candy bar, and bag of chips will be calling your name. If you're full, though, you lower the odds of succumbing to temptation. Fortunately, this isn't an eating plan that should leave you feeling hungry, thanks to the balance of nutrients that will maintain your blood-sugar levels all day long. Still, don't take that risk, and eat a meal or snack before heading to the store. It'll up your chances of sticking strictly to your list.

● **STAY SEASONAL:** Stick with seasonal and local products whenever possible, so you'll get produce when it's at its freshest, healthiest, and most flavorful. Nutrients begin to deteriorate as soon as fruits and veggies are harvested, but by eating locally, you minimize the amount of time needed to transport these foods. This is good news for your health, the environment, and for local farmers. Farmers' markets and produce stands are usually your best bet for finding fresh and seasonal products. Food co-ops are another good option. These member-run organizations often stock up on organic or pesticide-free produce, as well as local products. If none of these alternatives exist in your area, or if you just prefer the grocery store, don't hesitate to ask someone working at your supermarket to confirm which foods are in season. You can also visit the Natural Resources Defense Council to see what's in season in your state at nrdc. org/health/foodmiles. Keep in mind that frozen fruits and vegetables are packed at the peak of freshness and provide the same essential nutrients and health benefits as fresh, so if the fresh produce selection is skimpy, frozen produce (without added salt or sugar) is a good alternative.

● **START CLICKING:** If you really can't resist tossing that cake, box of cookies, or pint of ice cream into your shopping cart, there's always the Internet. Buying your groceries online is a good way to minimize impulse purchases. One study found that participants on weight loss plans who ordered groceries from online retailers stocked their kitchens with 28 percent fewer high-fat foods than those who shopped in their local grocery stores.[1] If you want to lessen the temptation and go online, you can try retailers such as Peapod (peapod.com), FreshDirect (freshdirect.com), or Amazon Fresh (fresh.amazon.com). And don't worry—you can still use your coupons on these Web sites. Another option is to check your local supermarkets to see if they offer delivery services. Some stores will do your shopping and deliver your groceries, while others will do the shopping and then you stop by to pick up your order. Either way, it keeps you away from temptation.

Get Savvy about Food Labels

To further enhance your supermarket know-how, it's important to be able to decipher the food labels you'll find on many of your favorite products. Grocery store shelves are full of foods that promise to boost your health and shrink your waistline, but what's actually good for you? To get beyond the promises, you need to look at the nutritional values, ingredients, and calorie counts of the foods you buy.

Though it might seem complicated at first, learning the basics of how food labels work can help you make the best food choices for you and your family. This will be especially important after these 2 weeks are over and you want to start creating your own healthy meals and snacks. Once you figure it out, the food label will become your best shopping tool. It allows you to compare the nutrients and ingredients in similar products, and it tells you which nutrients a particular food provides, and how much.

Most packaged products contain food labels, which you'll find on the back or side of the package. These labels contain an ingredients list, which lists ingredients in descending order by weight, as well as a "Nutrition Facts" panel. The panel lists the number of calories as well as how much total fat, saturated fat, trans fat, and other nutrients are in that food. There is also a column called "% Daily Value," which shows how much of the daily recommended nutrients the product provides, based on a 2,000-calorie diet. Some products also contain specific health claims, which must meet government regulations before they can appear on a package.

Here are some further tips to help you decode food labels:

● **SEEK THE REAL SERVING:** Don't forget to check the serving size of a product, which is also on the Nutrition Facts panel. All of the nutritional information you'll find on the label is based on this serving size. The label also tells you how many servings there are in the whole package.

This can be tricky, because a food that seems like a single serving (take a bagel or a bottle of soda) may be listed as two or three servings—and that means you'll get two or three times the calories if you consume the whole thing. Be sure to read the serving size information closely, so you know exactly what you're getting. Also, keep in mind that serving sizes aren't always reflective of the amount you should be eating of a particular food.

- **CALORIES STILL COUNT:** A food can be labeled as fat free, sugar free, low-fat, or low-carb, but still be unhealthy or high in calories. This is particularly true for healthier versions of junk foods, such as low-fat cookies, baked (rather than fried) potato chips, and reduced-fat ice cream or crackers. Sometimes, when a food's fat content is cut back, the amount of sugar or salt is increased to maintain flavor. That's not so healthy! Other times, low-fat foods have nearly as many calories as their original versions. So again, carefully check the Nutrition Facts panel to see how many calories per serving a product contains. And don't hesitate to compare the original version of a food with its "healthier" counterpart to get the full nutritional picture. Unfortunately, just because a food has a health claim doesn't automatically make it a healthy food.

- **GET THE WHOLE STORY:** Distinguishing a whole grain product from one that isn't can be difficult. Many breads, cereals, pastas, and other grain products have misleading names or package claims, for example "multigrain," which simply means that the food contains a variety of grains. It does not mean that the grains are whole. Instead, you want to go for foods with labels that say "100% whole grains" or "100% whole wheat." The best way to determine if a product is whole grain is to check out the ingredients list. The only grains in the list should be identified as whole: "whole wheat," "whole corn," or "whole rye." Of course there are exceptions, such as oat, buckwheat, and quinoa, which are also whole grains. If the ingredients list states "enriched flour" or "unbleached wheat flour," you'll know right away that the product contains some refined grains. It's also common to see wheat flour (white flour) as the first ingredient, followed by some sort of sweetener and then whole wheat flour, but this can mean that there's only a small amount of whole grain in the product.

- **TRACK TRANS FATS:** As you know by now, you want to avoid trans fats (also called trans fatty acids) at all costs, since they can be harmful to your heart. You'll find these bad guys most often in fried foods, some margarines, and commercial baked goods, such as cookies, crackers, and cakes. The good news is that these fats can now be found on the Nutrition Facts panel. As of January 2006, food manufacturers have been legally required

REAL 2-WEEK TURNAROUND SUCCESS STORY

Nancy Haley
2-WEEK RESULTS:
**7 pounds,
7¾ inches lost**

BEING PREPARED helped Nancy drop 7 pounds and more than 7 inches, including 2 inches off her waist. The day before she started her plan, Nancy went to the grocery store and bought almost everything she would need for the next 14 days. "I went online to *Prevention*'s My Health Tracker at prevention.com and planned out what I was going to eat. This way I had everything in the house. Those were my only choices, instead of it being a free-for-all foodfest whenever I wanted." Nancy uses another trick to stay on track—she stores her weights in a place in the kitchen where she can see them for motivation.

to list them. You'll find them listed directly under the line for saturated fat. Be aware, though, that even if the packaging says "no trans fats," the food can have up to 0.5 gram of trans fats per serving—and this can add up over time. What are other clues that a food contains trans fats? Look for the words "partially hydrogenated vegetable oil" in the ingredients list, as that's another term for trans fat. Often the words "vegetable shortening" is a good hint as it, too, contains some of these bad fats.[2]

● **LESS IS MORE:** Eating whole foods is about eliminating preservatives, additives, and processed sugars from your diet. It's about eating more fresh fruits and veggies, lean protein, low-fat dairy, and whole grains, and eating fewer processed foods with long lists of hard-to-pronounce artificial ingredients. Look for products with natural, real ingredients— things you can easily identify.

Get Cooking!

Once your kitchen is stocked with whole, healthy food options, you're finally ready to dig into the nutritionally balanced and mouthwatering recipes that make up this eating plan. Remember, healthy eating doesn't just happen because you buy all the "right" foods, you also need to prepare these foods in ways that retain their good-for-you properties. Whether you love spending time in the kitchen or prefer the quick route to a cooked meal, there are lots of small things you can do to boost the healthfulness of your dishes.

While we clearly lay out how to prepare the meals and snacks in this book, there are some additional cooking strategies you can use to boost the flavor and nutrition of the recipes. These tips and tricks will be especially important if you want to experiment with devising your own healthy meals once the 14 days are over. Don't forget, the cooking habits you form on this plan can be used for a lifetime. Here are some ideas to get you started:

● **PRESERVE NUTRIENTS:** How you choose to prepare your food can affect the amount of nutrients you end up eating. Some cooking methods are better than others, and you want to go for techniques that retain the most flavor, color, and nutrients in a food. So steam, stir-fry, or microwave veggies instead of boiling them, and avoid cooking at high temperatures or for extended cooking times. Too much liquid, heat, or time can destroy or leach out valuable nutrients.[3] Other healthy cooking methods include baking, grilling, and braising, while deep frying is really a no-no. Another trick is to use nonstick cookware, so less oil is necessary when cooking.

● **FLAVOR, MINUS THE FAT**: Using herbs and spices is an excellent way to boost flavor without increasing fat, calories, or salt. Fresh herbs work wonders, but the dried stuff is great, too. It's best to avoid prepared seasonings, as they often contain a lot of salt; otherwise, look for salt-free seasoning mixes. You can also make your own seasoning mix by blending together your favorite dried herbs. Other low-fat flavor-enhancers are lemon and lime juice, citrus zest, flavored vinegar, garlic, onions, and fat-free or low-fat sauces. If you really want to kick it up a notch, try adding hot chiles to your dish.

● **PREPARED PRODUCE**: Many people would be inclined to eat more health-boosting fruits and veggies if they weren't so short on time and overwhelmed by their busy schedules and lives. The good news is that in today's fast-paced world you can buy many of these products ready-to-eat—no chopping, no washing, no fuss. And they're usually just as nutritious as the unprepared version. So feel free to head to the produce section of your store and pick up prewashed salad and greens, as well as precut fruits and veggies. Just be sure to buy packages with no added sugar or salt, and if you're going for canned fruit, pick the ones packed in juice, not syrup. By keeping these easy-to-eat fruits and veggies on hand, you'll lower the odds of turning to unhealthy choices in a moment of hunger, and up the chances of filling your diet with these nutrient-dense superfoods.

● **CUT THE SALT**: Our bodies do need some sodium, which we mostly consume in the form of salt, to function properly. But eating too much sodium can increase your chances of developing high blood pressure, a condition that can lead to kidney disease. Since almost 80 percent of the sodium we eat comes from prepared or processed foods, you should skip these foods as much as possible, or choose sodium-free versions.[4] Herbs and spices, as you already know, are also a great way to cut the salt while maintaining the flavor. And be on the lookout for hidden sources of salt, such as bouillon cubes, marinades, soy sauce, and steak sauce (see page 21).

● **DEEP FREEZE**: If you're short on time or money, you'll be happy to know that frozen veggies are almost as good for you as the fresh stuff. Since you keep them in the freezer, they're also much less likely to go bad. It's true that just-picked produce has more vitamins and minerals, but these nutrient levels drop during shipping and storage. And most of our food travels a long way before it reaches the supermarket. In fact, most produce grown in the United States travels an average of 1,500 miles before it gets sold.[5] Frozen veggies, on the other hand, are usually picked ripe and then immediately flash frozen, so they retain most of their nutrients. To keep your calories under control, though, buy frozen veggies without added fat, and avoid those packed with salt, sauces, or additives. Also, stay away from canned veggies as much as possible, as they are often very high in sodium.

● **MAKE MEALS LAST:** Leftovers are your best friend when you're cooking healthy. If you're going to go through the effort, why not make a little extra? You can pack the leftovers for lunch the next day and voila!—you have a ready-made balanced meal. Or create your own frozen meal by freezing leftovers that you can pull out on busy days when you really don't have the energy to cook. When your stomach starts grumbling, heading to your freezer is a much better option than stopping by the nearest fast-food joint! To simplify things even further, separate your leftovers into smaller portions before putting them in the fridge or freezer. That way, when you—or a family member—reach in, you'll automatically grab one portion and be less likely to overeat. If you tend to forget about meals once they enter the freezer, keep a list on your fridge of the leftovers you've put away.

● **PORTION CONTROL:** Supersize meals and oversize dishes at restaurants have distorted our idea of a "normal" portion size. More often than not, we get more food than we need. Fortunately, you can avoid portion distortion at home. For starters, use small plates when dishing out homemade meals. Many of us instinctively clean off our plates, and a smaller plate translates into less food to polish off. It will also make the meal look larger. Another trick is to use the idea of a "divided plate."[6] Just think of the plate as being divided into four equal parts. Then fill one of the sections with a lean protein, such as chicken or fish, and another section with a starch, preferably a whole grain food. Finally, fill the remaining half of your plate with veggies. This will not only help limit how much you eat, but it will also keep your meals balanced.

All in the Family

Any journey to change old habits is easier if you don't go it alone. So make sure you give your family a heads-up that you're embarking on this eating plan. This will allow them to support you, provide motivation, and help you overcome any roadblocks as you attempt to stay on the healthy eating track. Our loved ones are often out biggest cheerleaders when we're trying to improve our lives, so take advantage of their encouragement.

At the same time, including your family on your healthy eating journey over the next 2 weeks may help them improve their eating habits. You can make a lasting positive impression, especially if you have younger kids, since they're impressionable and mostly eat what's available at home. If you junk-food-proof your house, the only options available when hunger strikes any member of your family will be whole and healthy foods. The best way to encourage your family to eat healthy is to do it yourself—this is your time to be a role model.

I realize this can be challenging, with everyone's busy schedules and varying tastes in food, not to mention the readily available unhealthy food options. But there are ways you can try to involve your family over the next 14 days. Here are some ideas:

PICK FAVORITES: Let your family help you choose which dinner recipes to include on some days of this eating plan. Most kids enjoy helping out with dinnertime decision making, and you can use this opportunity to talk to them about healthy food choices and planning a balanced meal. Your family will feel as if they're partaking in the eating plan as well, and they may be more inclined to eat dinner if they've been involved in the process. There are a multitude of delicious recipes in our eating plan, so it should be no problem finding meals you can all agree on. But don't let your kids dominate each day of this diet with their favorites, as kids need to develop a taste for new foods as well. And ultimately, this is *your* eating plan.

FAMILY MEALS: Schedule family meals several times during the week, if not every day. It will give your kids some structure and provide time for your family to reconnect and sample dishes from this meal plan together. Studies show that children who eat with their families tend to have healthier eating patterns. One study, part of the Project EAT-II research undertaken by the University of Minnesota's School of Public Health, showed that young people who ate more family meals during high school had better nutrition in their early years of adulthood. Specifically, they had a higher daily intake of fruit, vegetables, calcium, and other important nutrients, and a lower intake of soft drinks. Besides nutritional benefits, family meals have also been related to higher academic performance, greater psychosocial well-being, and a lower risk of unhealthy weight control behaviors, such as anorexia.[7]

SHOPPING TIME: It's true that taking the kids and your hubby along for grocery shopping can increase the amount of time spent at the store and probably raise the junk food content of your cart, but there are some advantages to bringing the family along. You can make the shopping list together and then tackle the list as a team once you hit the store. Once there, you can use the opportunity to teach your loved ones about healthy eating, healthy shopping, and how to read food labels. And don't stress if your family won't leave the store without a treat. It's not realistic to think that you'll eliminate all treats from your diet, especially if you stick to this plan for more than the 2 weeks. The key is to limit—not necessarily eliminate—the unhealthy foods in your diet, so one treat per person is fine.

Why not take your family along as you jump into this healthy eating plan? You never know, you may just help prepare them to make good food decisions in the process. That's not to say that suddenly your kids will want carrot sticks instead of potato chips, but the food habits you instill in them now can lead to healthier choices later in life.

Sampling Time

You now have all the tools you need to distinguish diet-sabotaging foods from health-boosting ones and to shop and cook in ways that will maximize your health. We're almost ready to launch into the recipes and meal plans in this diet. In the next four chapters you'll find tons of nutrient-dense breakfasts, lunches, dinners, snacks, and desserts. There's no way you won't find some new favorite meals in the upcoming chapters.

To get you started, here's a sample 2-week meal plan. Notice that it includes a balanced breakfast, lunch, and dinner, as well as an energy-boosting snack and a muscle-building snack. All of these recipes are delicious and good for you—you can't beat that!

MEAL GUIDELINES

Following these suggested amounts for each meal will help you organize your meals while staying on the eating plan.

BREAKFAST	A.M. SNACK	LUNCH	P.M. SNACK	DINNER
• 2 grains/starchy veggies • 1 dairy • 1 protein • 1 fruit • 1 fat	• 1 dairy • 1 fruit	• 1 grain/starchy veggie • 1 protein • 2 veggies • 1 fat	• 1 dairy	• 1 grain/starchy veggie • 1 protein • 2 veggies • 1 fat
(APPROXIMATELY 400 CALORIES)	(APPROXIMATELY 200 CALORIES)	(APPROXIMATELY 400 CALORIES)	(APPROXIMATELY 200 CALORIES)	(APPROXIMATELY 400 CALORIES)

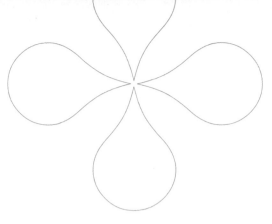

MEAL PLANS

DAY 1 Suggested Menu

BREAKFAST	SNACK	LUNCH	DINNER	SNACK
• Breakfast Pizza, page 59	• 1 part-skim string cheese with 1 cup grapes	• Warm Lentil Salad, page 107 • 1 cup pineapple chunks	• Turkey Cutlets with Mashed Sweet Potatoes, page 150	• Chocolate Pudding, page 223
PER SERVING: 388 calories; 18 g total fat; 4 g saturated fat; 38 g carbohydrate; 5 g fiber; 24 g protein; 18 mg cholesterol; 750 mg sodium	PER SERVING: 200 calories; 6 g total fat; 4 g saturated fat; 30 g carbohydrate; 1 g fiber; 8 g protein; 15 mg cholesterol; 150 mg sodium	PER SERVING: 441 calories; 16 g total fat; 3 g saturated fat; 59 g carbohydrate; 11 g fiber; 21 g protein; 23 mg cholesterol; 814 mg sodium	PER SERVING: 423 calories; 7 g total fat; 3 g saturated fat; 54 g carbohydrate; 7 g fiber; 36 g protein; 58 mg cholesterol; 491 mg sodium	PER SERVING: 166 calories; 4 g total fat; 1 g saturated fat; 29 g carbohydrate; 2 g fiber; 8 g protein; 3 mg cholesterol; 67 mg sodium

DAY 2 Suggested Menu

BREAKFAST	SNACK	LUNCH	SNACK	DINNER
• 1 cup whole grain flakes topped with 1 cup fat-free milk and 2 tablespoons sliced almonds. • Serve with 3 ounces lean meat (such as Canadian bacon) and ½ grapefruit.	• Stuffed Romaine Spears, page 246	• Mexican Chopped Salad, page 101	• ½ cup fat-free ricotta cheese topped with ¼ cup raisins and a sprinkle of cinnamon	• Grilled Whitefish with Edamame Pesto, page 190 • 2 cups sliced strawberries
PER SERVING: 450 calories; 13 g total fat; 2 g saturated fat; 67 g carbohydrate; 9 g fiber; 24 g protein; 19 mg cholesterol; 620 mg sodium	PER SERVING: 157 calories; 7 g total fat; 3 g saturated fat; 16 g carbohydrate; 3 g fiber; 10 g protein; 10 mg cholesterol; 203 mg sodium	PER SERVING: 386 calories; 18 g total fat; 3 g saturated fat; 26 g carbohydrate; 12 g fiber; 30 g protein; 64 mg cholesterol; 324 mg sodium	PER SERVING: 160 calories; 0 g total fat; 0 g saturated fat; 34 g carbohydrate; 1 g fiber; 6 g protein; 10 mg cholesterol; 70 mg sodium	PER SERVING: 434 calories; 15 g total fat; 2 g saturated fat; 44 g carbohydrate; 12 g fiber; 37 g protein; 65 mg cholesterol; 488 mg sodium

DAY 3 Suggested Menu

BREAKFAST	SNACK	LUNCH	SNACK	DINNER
• Quiche Cups Breakfast, page 61	• 1 cup vanilla soy milk with 1 peach	• Vegetable Fish Soup with Rouille, page 92 • 1 cup grapes	• 1 sliced pear with ¼ cup crumbled blue cheese	• Apricot Glazed Pork Skewers, page 178
PER SERVING: 412 calories; 11 g total fat; 4 g saturated fat; 34 g carbohydrate; 4 g fiber; 48 g protein; 198 mg cholesterol; 681 mg sodium	PER SERVING: 140 calories; 3 g total fat; 1 g saturated fat; 20 g carbohydrate; 1 g fiber; 7 g protein; 0 mg cholesterol; 170 mg sodium	PER SERVING: 423 calories; 8 g total fat; 1 g saturated fat; 64 g carbohydrate; 9 g fiber; 26 g protein; 49 mg cholesterol; 687 mg sodium	PER SERVING: 220 calories; 10 g total fat; 6 g saturated fat; 28 g carbohydrate; 6 g fiber; 8 g protein; 25 mg cholesterol; 470 mg sodium	PER SERVING: 425 calories; 11 g total fat; 1 g saturated fat; 44 g carbohydrate; 8 g fiber; 38 g protein; 74 mg cholesterol; 695 mg sodium

DAY 4 Suggested Menu

BREAKFAST	SNACK	LUNCH	DINNER	SNACK
• Swiss Muesli, page 79	• 1 apple with 1 slice (1 ounce) reduced-fat Cheddar cheese	• Turkey Grinder, page 118 • 1 large orange	• Shrimp Pasta Primavera, page 211	• Oatmeal Cookie with Warm Milk, page 233
PER SERVING: 379 calories; 7 g total fat; 1 g saturated fat; 53 g carbohydrate; 7 g fiber; 30 g protein; 0 mg cholesterol; 201 mg sodium	PER SERVING: 160 calories; 6 g total fat; 4 g saturated fat; 20 g carbohydrate; 3 g fiber; 6 g protein; 20 mg cholesterol; 240 mg sodium	PER SERVING: 406 calories; 4 g total fat; 1 g saturated fat; 72 g carbohydrate; 11 g fiber; 24 g protein; 25 mg cholesterol; 835 mg sodium	PER SERVING: 405 calories; 4 g total fat; 1 g saturated fat; 49 g carbohydrate; 5 g fiber; 38 g protein; 175 mg cholesterol; 423 mg sodium	PER SERVING: 207 calories; 5 g total fat; 1 g saturated fat; 31 g carbohydrate; 2 g fiber; 11 g protein; 5 mg cholesterol; 166 mg sodium

DAY 5 Suggested Menu

BREAKFAST	SNACK	LUNCH	SNACK	DINNER
• Cherry-Vanilla Smoothie, page 81	• Turkey Roll-Ups, page 245	• Salmon Salad, page 140	• Chilled Cucumber Soup, page 216	• Braised Beef with Greens and Bulgur, page 164
PER SERVING: 404 calories; 7 g total fat; 3 g saturated fat; 66 g carbohydrate; 5 g fiber; 22 g protein; 20 mg cholesterol; 377 mg sodium	PER SERVING: 203 calories; 9 g total fat; 4 g saturated fat; 9 g carbohydrate; 2 g fiber; 25 g protein; 45 mg cholesterol; 457 mg sodium	PER SERVING: 417 calories; 20 g total fat; 3 g saturated fat; 37 g carbohydrate; 7 g fiber; 24 g protein; 47 mg cholesterol; 433 mg sodium	PER SERVING: 191 calories; 8 g total fat; 4 g saturated fat; 20 g carbohydrate; 5 g fiber; 12 g protein; 17 mg cholesterol; 651 mg sodium	PER SERVING: 391 calories; 12 g total fat; 3 g saturated fat; 38 g carbohydrate; 11 g fiber; 34 g protein; 50 mg cholesterol; 615 mg sodium

DAY 6 Suggested Menu

BREAKFAST	SNACK	LUNCH	SNACK	DINNER
• Sweet Potato, Apple, and Sausage Hash, page 63 • 2 tablespoons almonds	• 1 cup low-fat or fat-free yogurt	• White Bean and Bulgur Salad, page 142	• Watermelon Feta Stacks, page 218	• Catfish Puttanesca, page 192
PER SERVING: 416 calories; 1 g total fat; 3 g saturated fat; 58 g carbohydrate; 12 g fiber; 24 g protein; 1 8 mg cholesterol; 611 mg sodium	PER SERVING: 140 calories; 0 g total fat; 0 g saturated fat; 19 g carbohydrate; 0 g fiber; 14 g protein; 4 mg cholesterol; 190 mg sodium	PER SERVING: 418 calories; 19 g total fat; 3 g saturated fat; 43 g carbohydrate; 11 g fiber; 20 g protein; 0 mg cholesterol; 609 mg sodium	PER SERVING: 182 calories; 10 g total fat; 6 g saturated fat; 16 g carbohydrate; 2 g fiber; 10 g protein; 28 mg cholesterol; 307 mg sodium	PER SERVING: 421 calories; 15 g total fat; 3 g saturated fat; 36 g carbohydrate; 6 g fiber; 35 g protein; 69 mg cholesterol; 549 mg sodium

DAY 7 Suggested Menu

BREAKFAST	SNACK	LUNCH	SNACK	DINNER
• Pumpkin Waffle, page 64 • 2 ounces cooked chicken and apple sausage • ¼ cup spiced applesauce • 1 cup fat-free milk	• Buffalo Celery Sticks, page 245	• Indian Spiced Turkey Wrap, page 120 • 1 cup sliced mango	• Slices from 1 orange dipped in 1 cup low-fat yogurt	• Chicken and Artichokes, page 208
PER SERVING: 381 calories; 9 g total fat; 2 g saturated fat; 53 g carbohydrate; 4 g fiber; 23 g protein; 45 mg cholesterol; 819 mg sodium	PER SERVING: 172 calories; 11 g total fat; 8 g saturated fat; 7 g carbohydrate; 2 g fiber; 11 g protein; 36 mg cholesterol; 584 mg sodium	PER SERVING: 432 calories; 5 g total fat; 1 g saturated fat; 64 g carbohydrate; 9 g fiber; 34 g protein; 71 mg cholesterol; 598 mg sodium	PER SERVING: 200 calories; 1 g total fat; 0 g saturated fat; 34 g carbohydrate; 3 g fiber; 15 g protein; 5 mg cholesterol; 190 mg sodium	PER SERVING: 415 calories; 8 g total fat; 1 g saturated fat; 47 g carbohydrate; 9 g fiber; 39 g protein; 66 mg cholesterol; 374 mg sodium

DAY 8 Suggested Menu

BREAKFAST	SNACK	LUNCH	SNACK	DINNER
• Breakfast Tostada, page 56	• Frozen Cinnamon Latte, page 240	• Ginger Broccoli Slaw with Tofu, page 117 • 2 cups almond milk • 1 tangerine	• 1 reduced-fat string cheese with 1 cup grapes	• Moroccan Shrimp Skewers, page 184
PER SERVING: 372 calories; 11 g total fat; 4 g saturated fat; 56 g carbohydrate; 6 g fiber; 18 g protein; 22 mg cholesterol; 545 mg sodium	PER SERVING: 202 calories; 0 g total fat; 0 g saturated fat; 44 g carbohydrate; 5 g fiber; 9 g protein; 5 mg cholesterol; 104 mg sodium	PER SERVING: 439 calories; 19 g total fat; 2 g saturated fat; 45 g carbohydrate; 11 g fiber; 24 g protein; 0 mg cholesterol; 874 mg sodium	PER SERVING: 200 calories; 6 g total fat; 4 g saturated fat; 30 g carbohydrate; 1 g fiber; 8 g protein; 15 mg cholesterol; 150 mg sodium	PER SERVING: 380 calories; 12 g total fat; 2 g saturated fat; 35 g carbohydrate; 11 g fiber; 36 g protein; 215 mg cholesterol; 530 mg sodium

DAY 9 Suggested Menu

BREAKFAST	SNACK	LUNCH	DINNER	SNACK
• Ricotta Pancakes, page 68	• Sweet Yogurt Dip, page 248	• Curry Chicken Salad Sandwich, page 122 • 2 tablespoons cashews	• Tabbouleh-Stuffed Portobellos, page 201	• Blueberry Lemon Pops, page 248
PER SERVING: 400 calories; 12 g total fat; 6 g saturated fat; 47 g carbohydrate; 5 g fiber; 28 g protein; 54 mg cholesterol; 810 mg sodium	PER SERVING: 205 calories; 3 g total fat; 0 g saturated fat; 28 g carbohydrate; 0 g fiber; 16 g protein; 0 mg cholesterol; 372 mg sodium	PER SERVING: 450 calories; 15 g total fat; 3 g saturated fat; 51 g carbohydrate; 17 g fiber; 42 g protein; 72 mg cholesterol; 266 mg sodium	PER SERVING: 326 calories; 6 g total fat; 1 g saturated fat; 48 g carbohydrate; 11 g fiber; 23 g protein; 4 mg cholesterol; 679 mg sodium	PER SERVING: 206 calories; 0 g total fat; 0 g saturated fat; 35 g carbohydrate; 2 g fiber; 18 g protein; 0 mg cholesterol; 73 mg sodium

DAY 10 Suggested Menu

BREAKFAST	SNACK	LUNCH	SNACK	DINNER
• Banana Smoothie, page 81	• Mini Pesto Pizza, page 247	• Grilled Vegetable Wrap, page 135	• Melon, Berry, and Brie Coupe, page 249	• Thai Noodle Bowl, page 199 • 2 tablespoons peanuts
PER SERVING: 397 calories; 7 g total fat; 1 g saturated fat; 68 g carbohydrate; 5 g fiber; 18 g protein; 3 mg cholesterol; 445 mg sodium	PER SERVING: 197 calories; 11 g total fat; 4 g saturated fat; 15 g carbohydrate; 3 g fiber; 12 g protein; 16 mg cholesterol; 425 mg sodium	PER SERVING: 373 calories; 15 g total fat; 2 g saturated fat; 41 g carbohydrate; 9 g fiber; 22 g protein; 0 mg cholesterol; 653 mg sodium	PER SERVING: 173 calories; 10 g total fat; 6 g saturated fat; 13 g carbohydrate; 2 g fiber; 9 g protein; 36 mg cholesterol; 240 mg sodium	PER SERVING: 432 calories; 21 g total fat; 5 g saturated fat; 44 g carbohydrate; 6 g fiber; 26 g protein; 0 mg cholesterol; 435 mg sodium

DAY 11 Suggested Menu

BREAKFAST	SNACK	LUNCH	DINNER	SNACK
• Whole Grain Waffle, page 80	• 1 apple with 1 slice (1 ounce) reduced-fat Cheddar cheese	• Turkey Chili Soup, page 84 • 2 cups cubed papaya	• Slow-Roasted Salmon with Tomato-Ginger Jam, page 181	• Raspberry Peaches with Greek Yogurt, page 249
PER SERVING: 397 calories; 4 g total fat; 2 g saturated fat; 68 g carbohydrate; 7 g fiber; 25 g protein; 12 mg cholesterol; 545 mg sodium	PER SERVING: 160 calories; 6 g total fat; 4 g saturated fat; 20 g carbohydrate; 3 g fiber; 6 g protein; 20 mg cholesterol; 240 mg sodium	PER SERVING: 430 calories; 8 g total fat; 1 g saturated fat; 64 g carbohydrate; 13 g fiber; 31 g protein; 41 mg cholesterol; 391 mg sodium	PER SERVING: 432 calories; 16 g total fat; 2 g saturated fat; 43 g carbohydrate; 7 g fiber; 29 g protein; 62 mg cholesterol; 451 mg sodium	PER SERVING: 222 calories; 1 g total fat; 0 g saturated fat; 35 g carbohydrate; 2 g fiber; 21 g protein; 0 mg cholesterol; 83 mg sodium

DAY 12 Suggested Menu

BREAKFAST	SNACK	LUNCH	SNACK	DINNER
• Stuffed Peach, page 79	• 1 cup low-fat yogurt	• Veggie Burger, page 145	• Apple Slices with Spiced Ricotta Dip, page 234	• Asian Fish Packets, page 212 • 2 kiwifruits
PER SERVING: 423 calories; 9 g total fat; 1 g saturated fat; 42 g carbohydrate; 4 g fiber; 49 g protein; 55 mg cholesterol; 591 mg sodium	PER SERVING: 140 calories; 0 g total fat; 0 g saturated fat; 19 g carbohydrate; 0 g fiber; 14 g protein; 4 mg cholesterol; 190 mg sodium	PER SERVING: 405 calories; 17 g total fat; 2 g saturated fat; 49 g carbohydrate; 13 g fiber; 18 g protein; 0 mg cholesterol; 695 mg sodium	PER SERVING: 225 calories; 4 g total fat; 1 g saturated fat; 32 g carbohydrate; 4 g fiber; 12 g protein; 20 mg cholesterol; 168 mg sodium	PER SERVING: 417 calories; 9 g total fat; 2 g saturated fat; 53 g carbohydrate; 8 g fiber; 35 g protein; 71 mg cholesterol; 494 mg sodium

DAY 13 Suggested Menu

BREAKFAST	SNACK	LUNCH	DINNER	SNACK
• Tofu and Sausage Breakfast Pocket, page 57	• 1 sliced pear with ¼ cup crumbled blue cheese	• Spinach Salad with Chicken Sausage, page 106 • 1 cup cherries	• Teriyaki Flank Steak with Shiitake Sauté, page 162	• Honeyed Yogurt Dip with Orange Sections, page 221
PER SERVING: 360 calories; 15 g total fat; 4 g saturated fat; 37 g carbohydrate; 9 g fiber; 24 g protein; 15 mg cholesterol; 488 mg sodium	PER SERVING: 220 calories; 10 g total fat; 6 g saturated fat; 28 g carbohydrate; 6 g fiber; 8 g protein; 25 mg cholesterol; 470 mg sodium	PER SERVING: 416 calories; 16 g total fat; 3 g saturated fat; 59 g carbohydrate; 13 g fiber; 19 g protein; 62 mg cholesterol; 708 mg sodium	PER SERVING: 387 calories; 14 g total fat; 3 g saturated fat; 32 g carbohydrate; 6 g fiber; 34 g protein; 37 mg cholesterol; 686 mg sodium	PER SERVING: 237 calories; 0 g total fat; 0 g saturated fat; 39 g carbohydrate; 4 g fiber; 21 g protein; 0 mg cholesterol; 85 mg sodium

DAY 14 Suggested Menu

BREAKFAST	SNACK	LUNCH	DINNER	SNACK
• Smoked Salmon Omelet, page 52	• Gorgonzola Dip with Crudités, page 246	• Spicy Sweet Potato Soup with Chicken, page 89 • 1 cup cubed honeydew melon	• Pork Chops with Apples and Collard Greens, page 173	• Vanilla and Orange Yogurt Cup, page 228
PER SERVING: 331 calories; 8 g total fat; 5 g saturated fat; 31 g carbohydrate; 6 g fiber; 34 g protein; 20 mg cholesterol; 773 mg sodium	PER SERVING: 168 calories; 6 g total fat; 4 g saturated fat; 14 g carbohydrate; 4 g fiber; 15 g protein; 17 mg cholesterol; 358 mg sodium	PER SERVING: 428 calories; 11 g total fat; 2 g saturated fat; 52 g carbohydrate; 10 g fiber; 30 g protein; 68 mg cholesterol; 366 mg sodium	PER SERVING: 406 calories; 13 g total fat; 3 g saturated fat; 42 g carbohydrate; 11 g fiber; 33 g protein; 66 mg cholesterol; 592 mg sodium	PER SERVING: 215 calories; 1 g total fat; 0 g saturated fat; 45 g carbohydrate; 5 g fiber; 9 g protein; 4 mg cholesterol; 132 mg sodium

CALORIE COUNTER

THE 2-WEEK TURNAROUND DIET is designed for you to eat three 400-calorie meals and two 200-calorie snacks daily. You'll find some of the recipes have fewer calories than the recommended amount. To round out these meals, always reach for nutrient-dense foods. Here are some easy ways to add around 100 calories to any recipe or meal.

For around 100 calories you can have . . .

- 2 tablespoons nuts
- 1 tablespoon peanut butter
- 1 slice whole grain bread
- 2 cups unsweetened almond milk
- 1 cup unsweetened soy milk
- 1 cup 1% or fat-free milk
- 1 part-skim string cheese
- ¼ cup raisins
- 1 cup pineapple chunks
- 1 cup grapes

- 1 cup sliced mango
- 2 kiwifruits
- 1 cup cherries
- 1 cup sliced pears
- 2 cups sliced strawberries
- 2 cups cubed papaya
- 2 cups cubed melon
- 1 banana
- 1 apple
- 1 orange

GROCERY LISTS

Following the suggested meal plan will be a breeze when your kitchen is stocked with all of the ingredients you'll need. Use the following lists to find everything necessary to prepare the recipes for the 2 weeks. Be sure to review the lists before heading to the market, checking off what's already in your kitchen. To make it easy for you to plan, we've listed the amounts by the typical package sizes you'll find in the store, as well as exactly how much you'll use each week if you follow our menus. This is especially important when shopping for week 2 because some of the ingredients purchased for week 1 will also be available for week 2.

STAPLES

- [ ] Canola oil
- [ ] Olive oil
- [ ] Toasted sesame oil
- [ ] Balsamic vinegar
- [ ] Seasoned rice wine vinegar
- [ ] White wine vinegar
- [ ] Low-fat Caesar salad dressing
- [ ] Low-fat Italian salad dressing
- [ ] Reduced-sodium teriyaki sauce
- [ ] Honey
- [ ] Maple syrup
- [ ] Dijon mustard
- [ ] Honey mustard
- [ ] Spicy brown mustard
- [ ] Parmesan cheese
- [ ] Garlic
- [ ] Ground cinnamon
- [ ] Ground cumin
- [ ] Ground ginger
- [ ] Italian seasoning
- [ ] Dried marjoram
- [ ] Dried oregano
- [ ] Paprika
- [ ] Hot-pepper sauce

- [ ] Black pepper
- [ ] White pepper
- [ ] Rubbed sage
- [ ] Salt
- [ ] Crab-boil seasoning
- [ ] Dried thyme
- [ ] Vanilla extract
- [ ] Baking powder
- [ ] Baking soda
- [ ] Cornstarch
- [ ] Cocoa powder
- [ ] Sugar
- [ ] Whole wheat pastry flour

WEEK 1 SHOPPING LIST

Breads

- [ ] 1 package (using 5) whole wheat flour tortillas (8″ diameter, about 120 calories each)
- [ ] 2 whole grain rolls (3 ounces each)
- [ ] 1 package (using 1) multigrain English muffins
- [ ] 1 8-ounce (using ½) whole wheat baguette

Produce

- [ ] 4 cups baby arugula
- [ ] 1 pound asparagus

- [ ] 1¼ pounds broccolini
- [ ] 1 pound (using 3) carrots
- [ ] 1 bunch (using 6 ribs) celery
- [ ] 2 ears corn
- [ ] 1 large (using 4½") cucumber
- [ ] 1 knob fresh ginger
- [ ] 6 cups frisée or mixed greens
- [ ] 1 small jicama
- [ ] 1 red onion
- [ ] 2 large sweet onions
- [ ] 2 onions (1 small + 1 medium)
- [ ] ¾ pound shiitake mushrooms
- [ ] 1 green bell pepper
- [ ] 3 large red or yellow bell peppers
- [ ] 4 small red potatoes
- [ ] 10 small romaine leaves or 2 romaine leaves and 8 endive leaves
- [ ] 1 bag (10 ounces) chopped romaine lettuce
- [ ] 7 scallions
- [ ] 4 large shallots
- [ ] 1 small bunch (using ¾ cup chopped) Swiss chard
- [ ] 2½ pounds sweet potatoes
- [ ] 4 tomatoes (1 large + 3 medium)
- [ ] 1 small zucchini
- [ ] 1 bunch basil
- [ ] 1 bunch (using 1 tablespoon chopped) chives
- [ ] 1 bunch cilantro
- [ ] 1 bunch mint
- [ ] 1 bunch parsley
- [ ] 1 container (using 1 teaspoon chopped) fresh oregano
- [ ] 1 container (using 1 teaspoon chopped) fresh thyme
- [ ] 4 apples
- [ ] 2 cups grapes

- [ ] 1 grapefruit
- [ ] 1 kiwifruit
- [ ] 1 cup sliced mango
- [ ] 1 cup cubed melon
- [ ] 2 large oranges
- [ ] 1 peach
- [ ] 1 pear
- [ ] 1 cup pineapple chunks
- [ ] 3 cups strawberries
- [ ] 8 ounces seedless, rindless watermelon
- [ ] 2 limes

Refrigerated Section

- [ ] 1½ dozen (using 4 whole eggs and 13 whites) eggs
- [ ] 1 4-ounce package (using ¼ + ⅓ cup) reduced-fat crumbled blue cheese
- [ ] 1 slice (1 ounce) reduced-fat Cheddar cheese
- [ ] 2 4-ounce packages (using 1 cup + 3 ounces) reduced-fat crumbled feta cheese
- [ ] 4 ounces low-fat goat cheese
- [ ] 1 8-ounce package (using 2 tablespoons) shredded reduced-fat Italian cheese blend
- [ ] 2 thin slices (1½ ounces) light Jarlsberg cheese
- [ ] 1 8-ounce package (using ¼ cup) shredded reduced-fat Monterey Jack cheese
- [ ] 1 8-ounce package (using ½ cup) shredded part-skim mozzarella cheese
- [ ] 1 8-ounce container (using ½ cup) fat-free ricotta cheese
- [ ] 1 8-ounce package (using 1) part-skim string cheese
- [ ] 1 16-ounce container (using 1 + ¾ cups) low-fat or fat-free Greek-style yogurt
- [ ] 1 16-ounce container low-fat yogurt
- [ ] 1 8-ounce container (using ¼ cup) reduced-fat sour cream
- [ ] 1 8-ounce package reduced-fat cream cheese

☐ 1 gallon (using 10½ cups) fat-free milk

☐ 1 quart (using 1 cup) low-fat buttermilk

☐ 1 quart (using 1 cup) fat-free half-and-half

☐ 1 quart (using 1½ cups) vanilla low-fat soymilk

☐ 1 12-ounce drained weight package (using 3 ounces) soft tofu, pureed

☐ 1 12-ounce drained weight package (using 3 ounces) firm low-fat silken tofu

☐ 1 8-ounce package (using 3 ounces) smoked tofu

Poultry, Meat, Fish

☐ 4 turkey cutlets (1 pound)

☐ 1¼ pounds 99% fat-free ground turkey breast

☐ 11 ounces thin-sliced natural low-sodium turkey breast from the deli

☐ 2 thick slices (2 ounces) natural low-sodium fat-free turkey breast

☐ 12 ounces boneless, skinless chicken breasts (using 3½ cups shredded)

☐ 1 pound chicken breast tenders

☐ 1 8-ounce package (using 1 link, 2 ounces) chicken and apple sausage

☐ 1 pound flank steak

☐ 1 pork tenderloin (using 8 ounces)

☐ 2 packages (6 ounces each) Canadian bacon

☐ 2¼ pounds cod, scrod, or other firm whitefish fillet

☐ 4 catfish or tilapia fillets (1¼ pounds)

☐ 1 4-ounce (using 3 ounces cooked) salmon

Pantry Items

☐ 1 package (32 ounces) reduced-sodium vegetable broth

☐ 1 14-ounce can (using ½ cup) reduced-sodium chicken broth

☐ 2 12-ounce boxes (using 16 ounces) whole grain penne pasta

☐ 1 10-ounce box (using ¼ cup) whole grain couscous

☐ 1 8-ounce bag (using 2 tablespoons) bulgur

☐ 1 9-ounce package (using 1¼ cups) whole wheat panko bread crumbs

☐ 1 12-ounce jar (using 3 peppers) roasted red peppers

☐ 1 can (14½ ounces) no-salt-added diced tomatoes

☐ 1 pound (using ¾ cup) green lentils

☐ 1 2-ounce can (using 3) anchovies

☐ 1 15-ounce can (using 1 cup) 100% pure pumpkin puree (not pie filling)

☐ 1 10-ounce jar (using 3 tablespoons) orange marmalade spreadable fruit

☐ 1 10-ounce jar (using ¼ cup) apricot spreadable fruit

☐ 1 9-ounce jar (using 2 tablespoons) prepared mango chutney

☐ 1 15-ounce can pinto or kidney beans

☐ 1 15-ounce can (using ¼ cup) reduced-sodium white beans

☐ 1 23-ounce jar (using ¼ cup) spiced applesauce

☐ 1 15-ounce box (using 1¾ cups) whole grain flakes cereal

☐ 1 18-ounce box (using ¾ cup) old-fashioned oatmeal

☐ 1 4-ounce package (using 2 tablespoons) pine nuts

☐ 12 kalamata olives from olive bar

☐ 1 15-ounce box (using ¼ cup) raisins

☐ 1 16-ounce jar (using ¼ cup) shelled peanuts

☐ 1 4-ounce bag (using ¼ cup) chopped walnuts

☐ 1 7-ounce bag (using 3 tablespoons) shelled unsalted pistachios

☐ 1 6-ounce bag (using 2 tablespoons chopped + 6) whole almonds

☐ 12 kalamata olives from olive bar

☐ 1 can cooking spray

Freezer Section

- [ ] 1 17.3-ounce box (using 1 sheet) puff pastry
- [ ] 2 packages (9 ounces each) frozen artichoke hearts
- [ ] 1 16-ounce bag (using 1 cup) frozen mixed bell peppers
- [ ] 1 bag (16 ounces) frozen broccoli, onions, mushrooms, and peppers
- [ ] 1 10-ounce bag (using 1½ cups) edamame
- [ ] 1 10-ounce package (using ¼ cup) frozen chopped spinach
- [ ] 1 package (16 ounces) frozen sugar snap peas
- [ ] 1 package (12 ounces) micro-steam sugar snap peas
- [ ] 1 16-ounce bag (using 1 cup) unsweetened frozen cherries
- [ ] 1 6-ounce can (using 2 tablespoons) frozen orange juice concentrate
- [ ] 1 box (6 ounces) soy breakfast sausage meat
- [ ] 1 pound frozen raw medium shrimp

WEEK 2 SHOPPING LIST

Breads

- [ ] 1 package (using 13) corn tortillas (6" diameter)
- [ ] 1 package (using 4) whole grain wraps or tortillas (8" diameter, about 120 calories each)
- [ ] 1 package (using 1) small whole wheat pita (4" diameter)
- [ ] 1 package (using 4½) large whole wheat pita (8" diameter)
- [ ] 1 package (using 1) whole grain or whole wheat English muffins
- [ ] 1 loaf (using 5 thick slices) whole grain bread

Produce

- [ ] 2 cups baby arugula or mixed greens
- [ ] 1½ pounds asparagus
- [ ] 1 (using ½) avocado
- [ ] 1 pound green beans
- [ ] 1 package (12 ounces) broccoli slaw
- [ ] 1 pound (using 4) carrots
- [ ] 2 6-ounce bags (using 5 cups) shredded carrots
- [ ] 1 bunch (using 2 ribs) celery
- [ ] 1 bunch (using 6 cups chopped) collard greens
- [ ] 2 (using 1½) pickling, or small, cucumbers
- [ ] 4 portobello mushrooms
- [ ] 1 package (8 ounces) sliced shiitake mushrooms
- [ ] 1 package (8 ounces) sliced white mushrooms
- [ ] 3 onions (2 medium + 1 large)
- [ ] 2 red onions (1 large + 1 small)
- [ ] 6 red bell peppers
- [ ] 1 small jalapeño chile pepper
- [ ] 6 medium russet potatoes
- [ ] 1 pound sweet potatoes
- [ ] 1 head (using 2 cups shredded) romaine lettuce
- [ ] 2 bunches (using 9) scallions
- [ ] 2 shallots
- [ ] 7 ounces snow peas
- [ ] 5 packages (7 to 9 ounces each) baby spinach
- [ ] 5 medium yellow squash (or mixture of yellow and zucchini)
- [ ] 24 large grape tomatoes
- [ ] 3 tomatoes
- [ ] 5 zucchini (4 medium + 1 small)
- [ ] 1 bunch basil
- [ ] 1 bunch cilantro
- [ ] 1 bunch mint

- [ ] 1 bunch parsley
- [ ] 1 bunch rosemary
- [ ] 1 knob (using 2 tablespoons grated) ginger
- [ ] 4 Golden Delicious or Granny Smith apples
- [ ] 1 small banana
- [ ] 2 cups blueberries
- [ ] ½ cup chopped cantaloupe
- [ ] 1 cup cherries
- [ ] 1 cup cubed honeydew melon
- [ ] 1 cup grapes
- [ ] 2 kiwifruits
- [ ] 3 lemons
- [ ] 2 limes
- [ ] 1 cup sliced mango
- [ ] 6 (using 5 whole oranges + 1 tablespoon juice and 2 teaspoons zest) navel oranges
- [ ] 2 cups cubed papaya
- [ ] 2 medium peaches
- [ ] 2 pears
- [ ] ½ pint (using ½ cup) fresh raspberries
- [ ] 1 pint strawberries
- [ ] 1 tangerine

Refrigerated Section

- [ ] 1½ dozen (using 13 whites) eggs
- [ ] 1 8-ounce container (using 2 tablespoons) reduced-fat sour cream
- [ ] 1 quart (using 3 cups) fat-free milk
- [ ] 1 4-ounce package (using ¼ cup) reduced-fat crumbled blue cheese
- [ ] 1 4-ounce piece (using ¼ cup cubed) brie cheese
- [ ] 1 slice (1 ounce) reduced-fat Cheddar cheese
- [ ] 1 8-ounce package (using 5 tablespoons) shredded reduced-fat Cheddar cheese
- [ ] 4 ounces (using ¼ cup crumbled) goat cheese

- [ ] 1 4-ounce package (using ⅓ cup) crumbled Gorgonzola cheese
- [ ] 1 8-ounce package (using 3 tablespoons) shredded part-skim mozzarella cheese
- [ ] 1 32-ounce container (using 15 ounces + 1 cup) fat-free ricotta cheese
- [ ] 1 part-skim string cheese
- [ ] 1 16-ounce container (using 1¾ cups) low-fat or fat-free plain yogurt
- [ ] 4 containers (16 to 17.6 ounces each) fat-free plain Greek-style yogurt
- [ ] 1 12-ounce drained weight package (using 3 ounces) soft silken tofu
- [ ] 1 12-ounce drained weight package (using 3 ounces) firm tofu
- [ ] 3 8-ounce packages (using 2½ packages) smoked tofu
- [ ] 1 7-ounce container (using 5 tablespoons) prepared reduced-fat basil pesto

Poultry, Meat, Fish

- [ ] 1 pound 99% fat-free ground turkey breast
- [ ] 1½ pounds boneless, skinless chicken breasts
- [ ] 1 package (12 ounces) chicken and apple sausage
- [ ] 2 6-ounce packages (using 9 ounces) Canadian bacon
- [ ] 1 flank steak (about 1 pound)
- [ ] 4 boneless pork chops (4 ounces each)
- [ ] 1¼ pounds large shrimp, peeled and deveined, with tails on
- [ ] 4 salmon fillets
- [ ] 4 tilapia fillets (1¼ pounds)
- [ ] 1 ounce thinly sliced smoked salmon

Pantry Items

- [ ] 4 ounces soba (buckwheat) noodles
- [ ] ¼ cup sun-dried tomatoes

- [ ] 1 can (15 ounces) kidney beans
- [ ] 1 can (15 ounces) petite diced tomatoes with basil and oregano
- [ ] 1 can (14½ ounces) reduced-sodium vegetable broth
- [ ] 2 packages (32 ounces each) reduced-sodium chicken broth
- [ ] 1 13.5- to 14-ounce can (using 1 cup) light coconut milk
- [ ] 1 32-ounce container (using 2 cups) almond milk
- [ ] 1 14-ounce box (using 1½ cups) long-grain brown rice
- [ ] 1 8-ounce bag (using 2½ cups) bulgur (cracked wheat)
- [ ] 1 3.52-ounce bag (using 12) caramel mini rice cakes
- [ ] 1 box (using 2 tablespoons) low-fat granola
- [ ] 1 10-ounce jar (using 2 tablespoons) raspberry spreadable fruit

- [ ] 1 16-ounce jar (using 2 tablespoons) shelled peanuts
- [ ] 1 4-ounce bag (using 2 tablespoons) cashews
- [ ] 1 6-ounce bag (using 6 tablespoons) sliced almonds

Freezer Section

- [ ] 1 6-ounce can (using 2 tablespoons) frozen orange juice concentrate
- [ ] 1 10-ounce box (using ¼ cup) frozen corn
- [ ] 1 9-ounce package (using 1) frozen whole grain low-fat waffle
- [ ] 1 10-ounce package (using 1) frozen veggie burger
- [ ] 1 12-ounce package (using 1 ounce) bulk soy sausage
- [ ] 2 6-ounce packages (using 7½ ounces) soy breakfast sausage links
- [ ] 2 6-ounce packages vegetarian sausage patties

CARB UP?

ARE YOU PLANNING TO inhale a pound of pasta to prepare for that 5K fun run? Think again. Carb loading involves increasing the amount of carbohydrates you eat for a few days before a high-intensity and long-duration athletic event, while decreasing your activity level. Done right, it can help build more glycogen (stored glucose) in your liver and muscles. Your body can then tap into this stored fuel once you start exercising, potentially boosting your performance.

But carb loading is necessary only if you're an endurance athlete taking part in activities that last 90 minutes or longer.[8] In fact, marathon runners and long-distance swimmers usually use this technique. The exercises in our workout plan don't require that level of physical intensity or last for such a long period of time.

That said, you can use some of the principles of carb loading even if you're not the next Lance Armstrong. Here's how it works: Take it easy for a day or two before your race or sporting event. Feel free to do some light exercise, but try to save your energy for the big day. The day before the event, make sure to drink lots of water and eat your normal balanced meals, such as the ones found in this eating plan. Keep in mind that it's best not to try any new foods just before a race. Hopefully these steps will help improve your performance!

BREAKFASTS

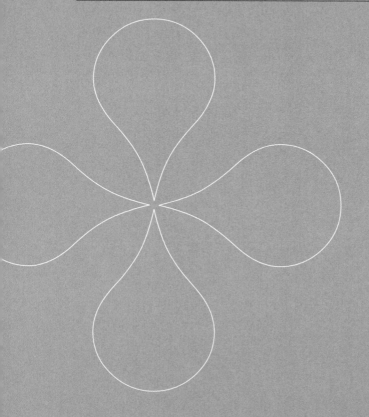

"IN THE LONG RUN, WE SHAPE OUR LIVES, AND WE SHAPE OURSELVES. THE PROCESS NEVER ENDS UNTIL WE DIE. AND THE CHOICES WE MAKE ARE ULTIMATELY OUR OWN RESPONSIBILITY."

—ELEANOR ROOSEVELT

SMOKED SALMON OMELET

5 egg whites

2 teaspoons chopped fresh parsley

⅛ teaspoon herbes de Provence, crushed

1 cup baby spinach

1 ounce thinly sliced smoked salmon

2 tablespoons (1 ounce) crumbled goat cheese

1 slice whole wheat bread, toasted

1 orange, sectioned

MADE IN MINUTES, omelets are a great last-minute meal, tasty any time of day. Omelets are also a clever use for cooked leftovers. In this recipe, you can replace the smoked salmon with leftover shredded chicken, coarsely chopped shrimp, or slivered fresh pork tenderloin. Replace the spinach with an equal amount of chopped vegetables, and the goat cheese with your favorite shredded cheese.

TOTAL TIME: 20 MINUTES

1. Whisk together the egg whites, parsley, and herbes de Provence in a medium bowl until blended. Set aside.

2. Heat a small nonstick skillet coated with cooking spray over medium heat. Cook the spinach in 1 tablespoon of water for 2 minutes or until wilted. Place in a bowl and set aside. Wipe the skillet clean.

3. Recoat the skillet with cooking spray and heat over medium heat. Add the egg mixture and cook, without stirring, for 15 seconds. When the edges begin to set, push them into the center with a rubber spatula, allowing the uncooked portion to cook. Cook for 2 to 3 minutes, continuing to the push edges into the center as they set, or until the eggs are no longer runny.

4. Scatter the spinach, salmon, and goat cheese on half of the omelet. Gently fold the other half over and cook for 1 minute to melt the cheese. Slide the omelet onto a plate. Serve with the toast and orange.

MAKES 1 SERVING

PER SERVING: 331 calories; 8 g total fat; 5 g saturated fat; 31 g carbohydrate; 6 g fiber; 34 g protein; 20 mg cholesterol; 773 mg sodium

NOTE: This recipe is a little high in sodium (you want to aim for no more than 600 to 650 milligrams per meal), so be sure to work this recipe into your daily total of 2,300 milligrams of sodium by selecting recipes for the remaining meals that are around 300 to 400 milligrams each.

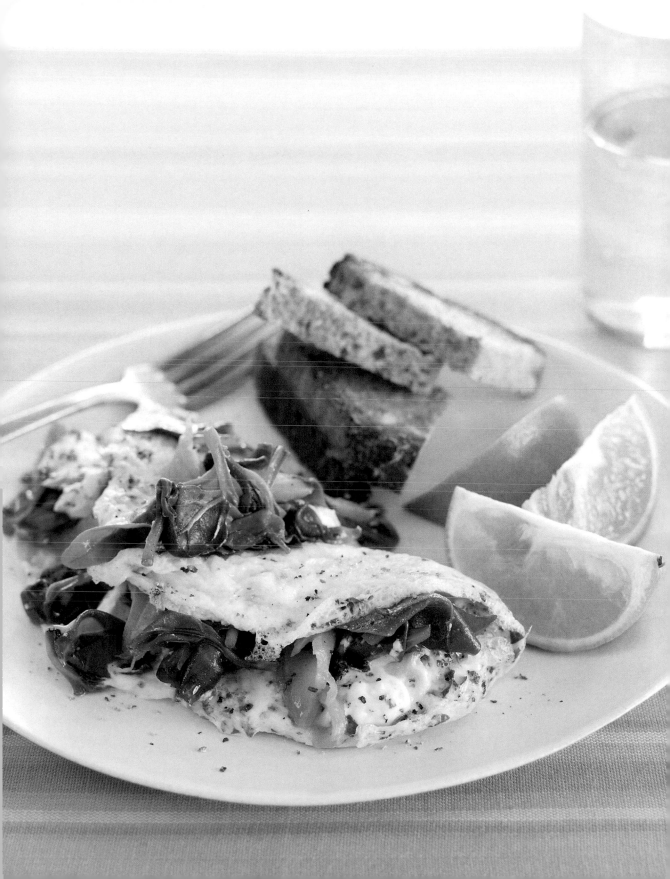

BROCCOLI STRATA CUPS

1½ cups frozen chopped broccoli (loose-pack), unthawed

2 scallions, chopped

1½ teaspoons Italian seasoning

4 ounces Canadian bacon, chopped

7 egg whites

½ cup 2% milk

¼ cup grated Parmesan cheese

1½ tablespoons dried bread crumbs

⅛ teaspoon freshly ground black pepper

½ cup shredded low-fat Swiss or sharp Cheddar cheese

2 whole wheat English muffins, toasted

¼ cup low-fat whipped cream cheese

4 plums, quartered

PERFECT FOR A Sunday brunch or a quick meal on the run, you can make these ahead and freeze them for up to 2 months. If you're feeling creative, mix some chopped fresh herbs into the whipped cream cheese for a flavorful spread.

TOTAL TIME: 45 MINUTES

1. Preheat the oven to 350°F. Coat a 12-cup muffin pan with cooking spray.

2. Heat a small nonstick skillet coated with cooking spray over medium heat. Add the broccoli and scallions and cook for 4 minutes, stirring occasionally. Stir in the Italian seasoning and cook for 1 minute or until the vegetables are just tender. Stir in the bacon and set aside to cool.

3. Whisk together the egg whites, milk, Parmesan cheese, bread crumbs, and pepper in a large bowl until blended. Stir in the broccoli mixture. Ladle ¼ cup of the mixture into each muffin cup. Divide the Swiss or Cheddar cheese evenly over the cups.

4. Bake for 20 minutes or until the cups are set in the center. To remove, run a narrow rubber spatula or knife around the edge of each muffin cup to loosen. Serve with the English muffins, spread with the cream cheese, and plums.

MAKES 4 SERVINGS (3 CUPS PER SERVING)

PER SERVING: 277 calories; 7 g total fat; 3 g saturated fat; 30 g carbohydrate; 5 g fiber; 25 g protein; 30 mg cholesterol; 832 mg sodium

NOTE: This recipe is a little high in sodium (you want to aim for no more than 600 to 650 milligrams per meal), so be sure to work this recipe into your daily total of 2,300 milligrams of sodium by selecting recipes for the remaining meals that are around 300 to 400 milligrams each.

PEPPER AND MUSHROOM FRITTATA

"THIS IS A delicious, healthy breakfast without a lot of work. I love making this for my family on the weekends. It has tons of flavor and protein."

TOTAL TIME: 15 MINUTES

1. Preheat the broiler. Beat the eggs, Parmesan cheese, and salt and black pepper to taste in a medium bowl.

2. Heat the oil in an ovenproof skillet over medium heat. Cook the bell pepper, onion, and mushrooms for 5 minutes, stirring occasionally, until lightly browned.

3. Pour the egg mixture into the skillet and cook for 4 minutes, or until the bottom has set and the top is starting to set.

4. Sprinkle with the parsley and broil for 3 minutes or until the top has started to brown.

5. Meanwhile, spread 1 teaspoon of the fruit spread on each piece of toast.

6. Cut the frittata into 4 wedges. Divide the wedges and toast among 4 plates.

MAKES 4 SERVINGS

PER SERVING: 298 calories; 16 g total fat; 5 g saturated fat; 20 g carbohydrate; 3 g fiber; 19 g protein; 427 mg cholesterol; 366 mg sodium

8 eggs

¼ cup grated Parmesan cheese

1 tablespoon olive oil

½ red bell pepper, chopped

½ onion, chopped

½ cup chopped mushrooms

¼ cup chopped parsley

4 teaspoons apricot all-fruit spread

4 slices whole wheat bread, toasted

BREAKFAST TOSTADA

1 corn tortilla

½ teaspoon canola oil

3 egg whites

2 tablespoons mild salsa, divided

1½ ounces soy breakfast sausage, chopped

¼ cup fresh or frozen and thawed corn

2 tablespoons shredded reduced-fat Cheddar cheese

1 to 2 tablespoons chopped cilantro

2 tablespoons reduced-fat sour cream

1 cup sliced mango

NOT JUST FOR breakfast, this flavorful meal is also great as a family lunch or dinner. Use any cooked chicken, pork, or shrimp leftovers in place of the sausage.

TOTAL TIME: 15 MINUTES

1. Preheat the oven to 400°F. Brush both sides of the tortilla with the oil. Place on a baking sheet. Bake for 6 to 8 minutes, or until crisp and golden.

2. Meanwhile, whisk the egg whites and ½ tablespoon salsa in a small bowl. Set aside. Heat a small nonstick skillet coated with cooking spray over medium heat. Cook the sausage and corn, breaking up with a spoon, for 3 minutes or until browned. Add the egg mixture and cook, stirring to scramble, for 1 to 2 minutes or until almost set.

3. Spread the mixture on the prepared tortilla and top with the cheese. Bake for 2 to 4 minutes, or until the cheese melts. Top with the remaining salsa, cilantro, and sour cream. Serve with the mango.

MAKES 1 SERVING

PER SERVING: 372 calories; 11 g total fat; 4 g saturated fat; 56 g carbohydrate; 6 g fiber; 18 g protein; 22 mg cholesterol; 545 mg sodium

METABOLISM BOOSTER: REV YOUR ENGINE

Caffeine not only perks up your mind, it can speed up your metabolism too. In fact, many researchers have looked closely at the caffeine–metabolism connection. One study found that people who drank caffeinated coffee with breakfast showed increased metabolic rates, compared to people who drank the decaffeinated option with breakfast.[1] There's more good news: People who drank caffeinated beverages reported being less hungry than those who didn't have these drinks.[2] And we all know that less hunger equals fewer reasons to give in to unhealthy cravings. However, caffeinated coffee and black and green teas are mild diuretics (they cause the body to lose water), so they should be limited to around 2 cups per day.

TOFU AND SAUSAGE BREAKFAST POCKET

S HORT ON TIME? Use 1 cup frozen mixed bell peppers and 1 teaspoon dried chives in place of the bell pepper and scallion. If you have a frozen sausage patty in your freezer, partially thaw, chop, and use it in place of the bulk sausage.

TOTAL TIME: 15 MINUTES

1. Heat the oil in a small nonstick skillet over medium heat. Add the bell pepper and cook, stirring occasionally, for 5 minutes or until softened. Stir in the sausage and scallion. Cook for 2 minutes or until browned.

2. Add the tofu, tarragon, and black pepper. Cook for 1 to 2 minutes, breaking up the tofu and stirring frequently until heated through. Stir in the cheese until melted.

3. Spoon into the pita and serve with the strawberries.

MAKES 1 SERVING

PER SERVING: 360 calories; 15 g total fat; 4 g saturated fat; 37 g carbohydrate; 9 g fiber; 24 g protein; 15 mg cholesterol; 488 mg sodium

1 teaspoon olive oil

½ red bell pepper, chopped

1 ounce bulk soy sausage (2 tablespoons or one 2½" slice), crumbled

1 large scallion, chopped

2 ounces firm tofu, drained

¼ teaspoon dried tarragon, crumbled

Pinch freshly ground black pepper

3 tablespoons shredded reduced-fat Cheddar cheese

½ whole wheat pita

1 cup strawberries

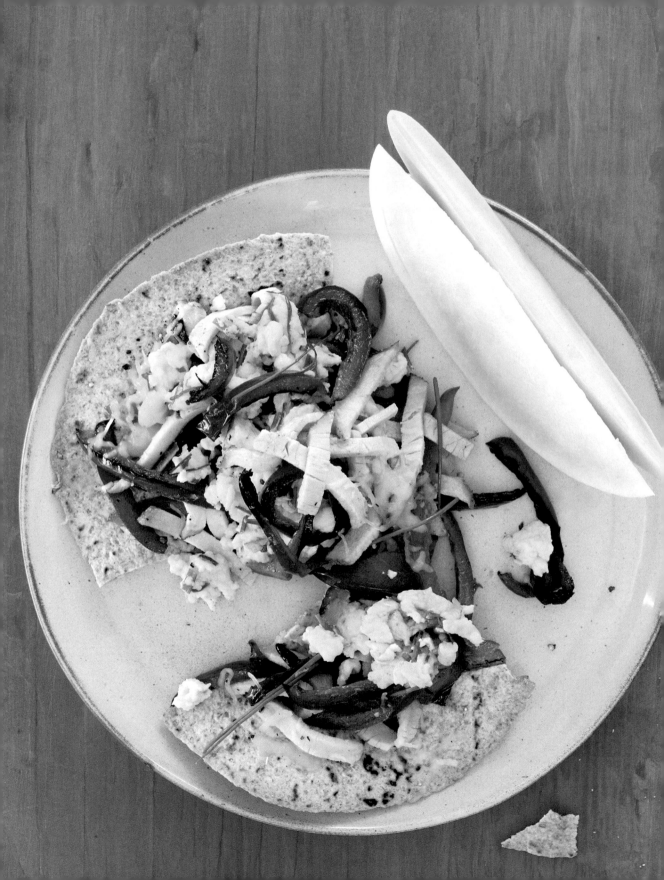

BREAKFAST PIZZA

YOU CAN ALSO turn this pizza into a lunchtime treat by replacing the egg with ¼ cup prepared low-fat tomato meat sauce. Round out the meal with some carrot and celery sticks.

TOTAL TIME: 25 MINUTES

1. Preheat the oven to 400°F. Coat both sides of the tortilla with cooking spray and place on a baking sheet. Bake for 6 minutes or until golden and crisp.

2. Meanwhile, heat the oil in a small nonstick skillet over medium heat. Cook the pepper for 5 minutes or until tender. Place on a plate.

3. Beat the egg whites, chives, oregano, and 2 teaspoons water in a medium bowl. Pour into the same skillet and cook over medium heat, stirring to scramble, for 2 minutes or until almost set.

4. Scatter about two-thirds of the pepper and bacon strips on the tortilla. Top with the cooked eggs, remaining pepper and bacon strips, and cheese. Bake for 4 minutes or until the cheese is melted. Cut into fourths and serve with the melon.

MAKES 1 SERVING

PER SERVING: 388 calories; 18 g total fat; 4 g saturated fat; 38 g carbohydrate; 5 g fiber; 24 g protein; 18 mg cholesterol; 750 mg sodium

NOTE: This recipe is a little high in sodium (you want to aim for no more than 600 to 650 milligrams per meal), so be sure to work this recipe into your daily total of 2,300 milligrams of sodium by selecting recipes for the remaining meals that are around 300 to 400 milligrams each.

1 whole wheat flour tortilla (8″ diameter)

1 tablespoon olive oil

½ red bell pepper, cut into thin strips

3 egg whites

1 tablespoon chopped chives

1 teaspoon chopped fresh oregano or ½ teaspoon dried

1 ounce Canadian bacon, cut into thin strips

2 tablespoons shredded reduced-fat Italian cheese blend

1 cup cubed melon or 2 thin wedges (about ⅛ of a melon)

CHAPTER 4 ○ BREAKFASTS

SAUSAGE AND APPLE STRATA

2 apples, peeled, cored, and coarsely chopped

12 ounces Turkey Breakfast Sausage (page 62)

2 whole grain English muffins, cut in ½" pieces

3 scallions, chopped

¼ cup + 2 tablespoons shredded low-fat Swiss cheese

2 cups fat-free milk

8 egg whites

2 tablespoons grated Parmesan cheese

½ teaspoon dry mustard

¼ teaspoon freshly ground black pepper

PREPARE THIS MAKE-AHEAD casserole the night before for an effortless breakfast, or double the recipe for a Sunday brunch gathering. If you have leftovers, they warm perfectly in the microwave. Serve with a crisp green salad for a weekend lunch.

TOTAL TIME: 1 HOUR, 10 MINUTES, PLUS CHILLING/STANDING TIME

1. Coat a 2-quart (9" x 9") baking dish with cooking spray. Place the apples in a microwaveable bowl and cover. Microwave on high for 3 minutes; uncover to cool.

2. Heat a nonstick skillet coated with cooking spray over medium-low heat. Crumble the sausage and cook for 2 to 3 minutes or until golden brown and cooked through. Scatter the apples, sausage, muffins, scallions, and Swiss cheese in the bottom of the dish.

3. Whisk together the milk, egg whites, Parmesan cheese, mustard, and pepper in a large bowl. Pour evenly over the ingredients in the casserole. Cover with plastic and refrigerate for 1 to 12 hours.

4. Preheat the oven to 375°F. Bake for 50 to 55 minutes or until a knife inserted in the center comes out clean. Let stand for 15 minutes and serve hot or warm.

MAKES 4 SERVINGS

PER SERVING: 307 calories; 3 g total fat; 1 g saturated fat; 35 g carbohydrate; 4 g fiber; 37 g protein; 70 mg cholesterol; 510 mg sodium

QUICHE CUPS

"THESE QUICHE CUPS are great for entertaining! They look amazing with a little garnish. Perfect for brunch. Have any leftovers? No problem, they keep well for a few days stored in the refrigerator in a sealed container. Simply pop in the microwave for a great quick meal in no time."

TOTAL TIME: 45 MINUTES

1. Preheat the oven to 350°F. Coat a 12-cup muffin pan with cooking spray.
2. Unfold the puff pastry and cut into 12 equal squares. Place one square in each muffin cup and pierce the bottom with a fork.
3. Whisk together the eggs, half-and-half, Parmesan cheese, mozzarella cheese, tomatoes, spinach, and pepper in a medium bowl.
4. Divide the egg mixture among the muffin cups.
5. Bake for 35 minutes or until a knife inserted in the center comes out clean. Serve warm or cold.

MAKES 6 SERVINGS

PER SERVING: 149 calories; 9 g total fat; 4 g saturated fat; 8 g carbohydrate; 1 g fiber; 10 g protein; 150 mg cholesterol; 250 mg sodium

1 sheet frozen puff pastry, thawed

4 eggs

1 cup fat-free half-and-half

¼ cup shredded Parmesan cheese

½ cup shredded part-skim mozzarella cheese

2 medium tomatoes, chopped

¼ cup frozen chopped spinach, thawed and squeezed dry

¼ teaspoon black pepper

Quiche Cups Breakfast

Serve 2 quiche cups (1 serving) with 2 Turkey Breakfast Sausage patties (page 62), 1 cup fat-free milk, and 1 cup strawberries.

MAKES 1 SERVING

PER SERVING: 412 calories; 11 g total fat; 4 g saturated fat; 34 g carbohydrate; 4 g fiber; 48 g protein; 198 mg cholesterol; 681 mg sodium

NOTE: This recipe is a little high in sodium (you want to aim for no more than 600 to 650 milligrams per meal), so be sure to work this recipe into your daily total of 2,300 milligrams of sodium by selecting recipes for the remaining meals that are around 300 to 400 milligrams each.

TURKEY SAUSAGE

½ small onion, grated

2 tablespoons chopped parsley

1½ teaspoons paprika

¾ teaspoon rubbed sage

¼ teaspoon ground ginger

¼ teaspoon marjoram or oregano, crumbled

½ teaspoon salt

¾ teaspoon freshly ground black pepper

1¼ pounds 99% fat-free ground turkey breast

PERFECT TO HAVE at the ready, you can shape this sausage meat into patties or logs and freeze up to 2 months in advance. Use the patties for a quick breakfast sandwich, or crumble the bulk sausage to use in the Sweet Potato, Apple, and Sausage Hash (opposite), Sausage and Apple Strata (page 60), or Tofu and Sausage Breakfast Pocket (page 57) recipes.

TOTAL TIME: 20 MINUTES PLUS CHILLING TIME

1. Stir together the onion, parsley, paprika, sage, ginger, marjoram or oregano, salt, and pepper in a large bowl. Add the turkey and stir until well blended.

2. To shape into logs: Divide the mixture in half and spoon onto 2 sheets of plastic wrap. Wrap in the plastic wrap, twisting the ends. Roll on the countertop to shape into logs, about 2″ in diameter. Freeze for 1 hour or until slightly firm. (Can be refrigerated overnight.)

3. To shape into patties: Use 2 slightly rounded tablespoonfuls of the mixture for each patty. Shape into rounds, 2″ in diameter. To freeze, place patties on a plastic-lined baking sheet in the freezer for 1 hour or until firm. Transfer to a food storage bag, seal, and freeze.

4. To cook, slice each log into 5 rounds. Heat a large nonstick skillet coated with cooking spray over medium-low heat. Cook the patties for 3 to 4 minutes per side or until golden brown and cooked through.

MAKES 5 SERVINGS (2 PATTIES EACH)

PER SERVING: 127 calories; 2 g total fat; 0 g saturated fat; 1 g carbohydrate; 0 g fiber; 28 g protein; 45 mg cholesterol; 299 mg sodium

● Turkey Sausage Breakfast

Cook 2 turkey sausage patties. Divide 1 multigrain English muffin in half and toast the bottoms under the broiler for 2 minutes. Turn over and top each half with 2 tablespoons shredded low-fat Swiss cheese. Broil for 2 minutes or until the cheese melts. Serve with the sausage and 1 small apple.

MAKES 1 SERVING

PER SERVING: 403 calories; 5 g total fat; 1 g saturated fat; 55 g carbohydrate; 8 g fiber; 41 g protein; 54 mg cholesterol; 541 mg sodium

SWEET POTATO, APPLE, AND SAUSAGE HASH

FEEL FREE TO substitute an equal weight of chopped Canadian bacon for the sausage. If you find yourself with leftovers, this hash will reheat nicely in the microwave or a small nonstick skillet.

TOTAL TIME: 25 MINUTES

1. Place the potato and 1 tablespoon water in a microwaveable bowl. Cover and microwave on high for 4 minutes or until just tender. Drain well.

2. Meanwhile, heat a large nonstick skillet coated with cooking spray over medium heat. Cook the sausage for 4 minutes or until browned, breaking up the meat with the side of a spoon.

3. Add the bell peppers and apple and cook, stirring occasionally, for 6 minutes or until tender-crisp.

4. Stir in the potato, scallions, parsley, thyme, black pepper, and sage. Cook, stirring occasionally, for 4 to 6 minutes or until golden. Sprinkle with the cheese, cover, and remove from the heat. Let stand for 5 minutes or until the cheese is just melted.

MAKES 2 SERVINGS

PER SERVING: 317 calories; 3 g total fat; 2 g saturated fat; 54 g carbohydrate; 10 g fiber; 20 g protein; 8 mg cholesterol; 611 mg sodium

1 large sweet potato (8 ounces), peeled and cut into ½" cubes

6 ounces soy breakfast sausage meat

1 cup frozen mixed bell peppers

1 large apple, peeled, cored, and diced

2 scallions, chopped

2 tablespoons chopped fresh parsley

1½ teaspoons chopped fresh thyme (or ½ teaspoon dried thyme)

¼ teaspoon black pepper

⅛ teaspoon ground sage

¼ cup shredded reduced-fat Monterey Jack cheese

PUMPKIN WAFFLES

5 egg whites

1½ cups whole wheat pastry flour

2 teaspoons baking powder

1 teaspoon baking soda

2 teaspoons cinnamon

¼ teaspoon salt

½ cup low-fat soy milk

1 cup canned 100% pure pumpkin puree (not pie filling)

4 tablespoons honey

2 tablespoons canola oil

1 teaspoon vanilla extract

A MARVELOUS MAKE-AHEAD MEAL, leftover waffles can be individually wrapped and frozen for up to 2 months. To reheat, simply pop in a toaster or toaster oven for a quick breakfast treat.

TOTAL TIME: 35 MINUTES

1. Coat a nonstick waffle iron with cooking spray. Preheat according to the manufacturer's directions.

2. Place the egg whites in a mixing bowl and beat on high until stiff peaks form.

3. Whisk together the flour, baking powder, baking soda, cinnamon, and salt in a medium bowl. Whisk in the soy milk, pumpkin, honey, oil, and vanilla just until blended. Gently fold in the egg whites until just combined.

4. Spoon ½ cup of batter on the bottom grids, covering two-thirds of the grids. Close the iron and bake according to the manufacturer's directions.

5. Using a rubber spatula, carefully remove the waffle from the iron. Repeat with the remaining batter.

MAKES 8 WAFFLES

PER WAFFLE: 165 calories; 4 g total fat; 0 g saturated fat; 27 g carbohydrate; 3 g fiber; 5 g protein; 0 mg cholesterol; 395 mg sodium

● Pumpkin Waffle Breakfast

Serve 1 pumpkin waffle with 1 teaspoon maple syrup; 2 ounces cooked chicken and apple sausage; ½ small apple, sliced; and 1 cup fat-free milk.

MAKES 1 SERVING

PER SERVING: 411 calories; 9 g total fat; 2 g saturated fat; 60 g carbohydrate; 5 g fiber; 23 g protein; 45 mg cholesterol; 819 mg sodium

NOTE: This recipe is a little high in sodium (you want to aim for no more than 600 to 650 milligrams per meal), so be sure to work this recipe into your daily total of 2,300 milligrams of sodium by selecting recipes for the remaining meals that are around 300 to 400 milligrams each.

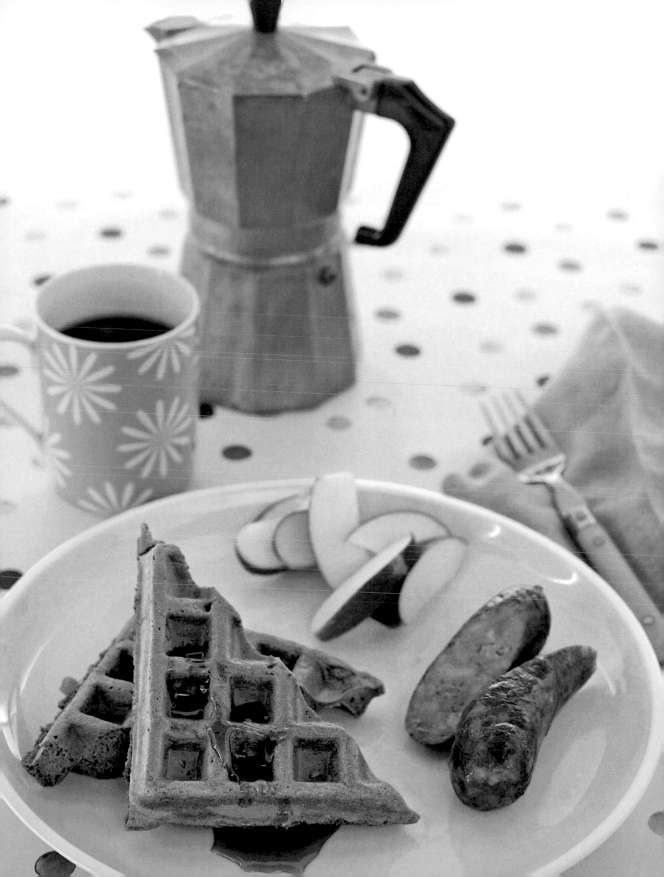

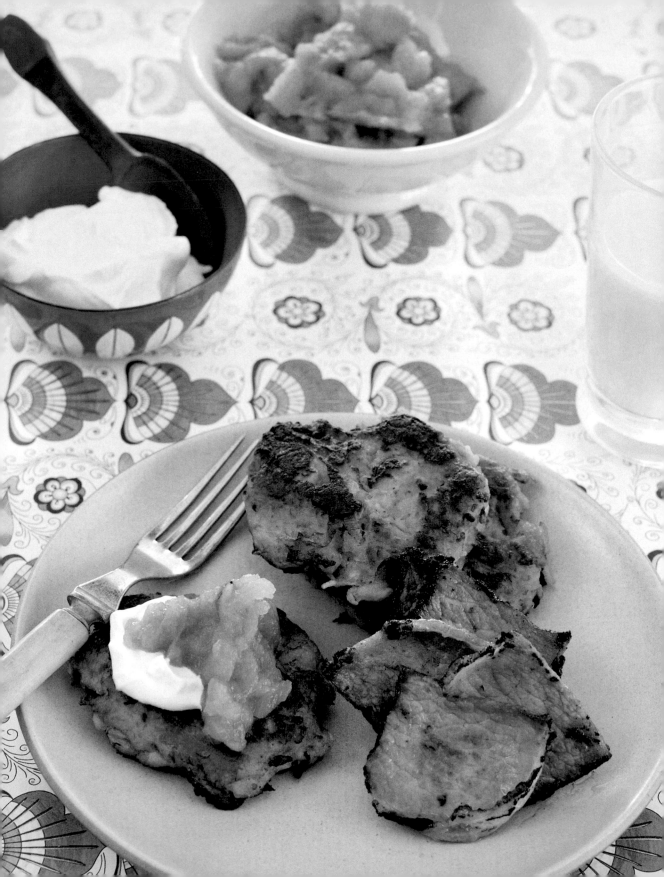

SWEET POTATO PANCAKES

FOR A LITTLE variety, try substituting shredded parsnips or Yukon gold potatoes for half of the sweet potatoes. You can also double the recipe, refrigerate the leftovers, and warm in a skillet to serve.

TOTAL TIME: 35 MINUTES

1. Steam the potato in a steamer set in a pan of boiling water for 12 to 15 minutes or until very tender. Place in a large bowl and mash until almost smooth. Add the scallions, egg whites, pepper, and nutmeg and mash to combine.

2. Heat a nonstick skillet coated with cooking spray over medium heat. Add 1 teaspoon of the oil until hot. Drop the potato mixture into the skillet, using ¼ cup for each of 3 pancakes. Flatten mounds into 3″ rounds. Cook, turning once, for 6 to 8 minutes or until golden brown. Transfer to a plate; cover to keep warm. Repeat with the remaining oil and potato mixture to make 6 pancakes.

3. Add the bacon to the skillet and cook for 2 to 4 minutes, turning once, or until heated through. Serve the pancakes with the bacon, applesauce, and sour cream. Serve with 1 cup of fat-free milk each.

MAKES 2 SERVINGS

PER SERVING: 385 calories; 10 g total fat; 3 g saturated fat; 52 g carbohydrate; 5 g fiber; 23 g protein; 31 mg cholesterol; 757 mg sodium

NOTE: This recipe is a little high in sodium (you want to aim for no more than 600 to 650 milligrams per meal), so be sure to work this recipe into your daily total of 2,300 milligrams of sodium by selecting recipes for the remaining meals that are around 300 to 400 milligrams each.

1 large sweet potato (12 ounces), peeled and cubed

2 scallions, chopped

2 egg whites

⅛ teaspoon ground black pepper

Pinch grated nutmeg

2 teaspoons canola oil, divided

4 ounces Canadian bacon

1 cup unsweetened applesauce

2 tablespoons reduced-fat sour cream

2 cups fat-free milk

CHAPTER 4 ∘ BREAKFASTS

RICOTTA PANCAKES

8 ounces Canadian bacon

4 navel oranges

1 container (15 ounces) part-skim ricotta

5 egg whites

3 tablespoons agave nectar or honey, divided

½ cup whole wheat pastry flour

½ teaspoon baking powder

THE MINIMAL AMOUNT of flour in this recipe results in super-moist, richly ricotta-flavored pancakes. This batter is easily halved, if you're cooking for 2. For a delicious dessert, top 2 pancakes with a berry compote.

TOTAL TIME: 20 MINUTES

1. Preheat the oven to 300°F. Place the bacon in a single layer on a small foil-lined pan; cover with foil.

2. Grate 2 teaspoons of zest from one orange. Cut off the peel and pith of oranges and discard. Cut the fruit into segments and place in a medium bowl.

3. Whisk together the ricotta, egg whites, 1 tablespoon of agave nectar or honey, and orange zest in a large bowl until blended. Sprinkle the flour and baking powder over the mixture. Stir just until blended.

4. Heat the bacon in the oven for 12 minutes or until heated through.

5. Meanwhile, heat a large nonstick skillet coated with cooking spray over medium heat. Drop the batter by 2 tablespoonfuls (slightly rounded), shaping into 3" rounds. Cook for 3 to 4 minutes per side, or until golden.

6. Divide the pancakes, Canadian bacon, and oranges among 4 plates. Drizzle the pancakes with the remaining 2 tablespoons of agave nectar or honey.

MAKES 4 SERVINGS

PER SERVING: 400 calories; 12 g total fat; 6 g saturated fat; 47 g carbohydrate; 5 g fiber; 28 g protein; 54 mg cholesterol; 810 mg sodium

NOTE: This recipe is a little high in sodium (you want to aim for no more than 600 to 650 milligrams per meal), so be sure to work this recipe into your daily total of 2,300 milligrams of sodium by selecting recipes for the remaining meals that are around 300 to 400 milligrams each.

SPICY CARROT MUFFINS

"I HAVE ALWAYS BEEN a lover of spice-cake-type desserts, so I came up with this healthier option to satisfy my sweet tooth. I sometimes enjoy these muffins along with yogurt and fruit for a hearty breakfast."

TOTAL TIME: 40 MINUTES

1. Preheat the oven to 375°F. Coat a 12-cup muffin pan with cooking spray or line with paper liners.
2. Whisk together the flour, sugar, baking powder, baking soda, cinnamon, salt, nutmeg, and ginger in a large bowl.
3. Stir together the carrots, yogurt, butter, milk, egg, and vanilla in a medium bowl. Stir into the flour mixture just until blended.
4. Divide the batter into the muffin cups. Bake for 18 to 20 minutes or until a wooden pick inserted in the center comes out clean. Let cool in the pan for 5 minutes. Remove to a rack to cool completely.

MAKES 12 MUFFINS

PER MUFFIN: 161 calories; 5 g total fat; 3 g saturated fat; 27 g carbohydrate; 2 g fiber; 4 g protein; 29 mg cholesterol; 345 mg sodium

1¾ cups whole grain pastry flour

¾ cup packed brown sugar

2 teaspoons baking powder

1 teaspoon baking soda

1 teaspoon ground cinnamon

½ teaspoon salt

½ teaspoon ground nutmeg

¼ teaspoon ground ginger

1¾ cups shredded carrots

¾ cup low-fat plain yogurt

¼ cup butter, melted

¼ cup fat-free milk

1 egg

1 teaspoon vanilla extract

CHAPTER 4 ○ BREAKFASTS

● Spicy Carrot Muffin Breakfast

Serve 1 muffin with 1 serving cooked Turkey Sausage Breakfast (page 62) and 1 cup fat-free milk.

MAKES 1 SERVING

PER SERVING: 379 calories; 6 g total fat; 3 g saturated fat; 42 g carbohydrate; 2 g fiber; 41 g protein; 77 mg cholesterol; 774 mg sodium

NOTE: This recipe is a little high in sodium (you want to aim for no more than 600 to 650 milligrams per meal), so be sure to work this recipe into your daily total of 2,300 milligrams of sodium by selecting recipes for the remaining meals that are around 300 to 400 milligrams each.

HOMEMADE GRANOLA

2 cups old-fashioned oats

2 tablespoons packed brown sugar

2 tablespoons honey

2 teaspoons canola oil

1 teaspoon vanilla extract

½ teaspoon ground cinnamon

⅛ teaspoon salt

1 tablespoon ground flaxseed

¼ cup roasted soy nuts or sunflower seeds

GREAT TO HAVE on hand, use a sprinkling of this granola to top off fresh fruit or yogurt. If you like, double up this recipe and divide between 2 jelly-roll pans. Bake as directed, rotating the pans in the oven (switching from top to bottom) halfway during the cooking.

TOTAL TIME: 45 MINUTES PLUS COOLING TIME

1. Preheat the oven to 350°F.
2. Spread the oats in a single layer on a jelly-roll pan. Bake for 18 minutes or until toasted, stirring halfway through the cooking time.
3. Meanwhile, whisk together the sugar, honey, oil, vanilla, cinnamon, and salt in a large bowl until blended. Toss in the hot oats until evenly coated.
4. Coat the same pan with cooking spray. Spread the granola in an even layer. Bake for 13 to 15 minutes or until golden brown. Sprinkle the flaxseed evenly on top. Cool in the pan on a rack for 30 minutes. Stir in the soy nuts or sunflower seeds. Store in an airtight container.

MAKES 6 SERVINGS

PER SERVING: 187 calories; 5 g total fat; 0 g saturated fat; 30 g carbohydrate; 3 g fiber; 6 g protein; 0 mg cholesterol; 64 mg sodium

● Homemade Granola Breakfast

Combine ½ cup granola, 1 cup fat-free yogurt, and 1 peach, cut into wedges, in a small bowl.

MAKES 1 SERVING

PER SERVING: 347 calories; 5 g total fat; 0 g saturated fat; 64 g carbohydrate; 5 g fiber; 17 g protein; 5 mg cholesterol; 199 mg sodium

GRANOLA BAKED APPLES

CHOOSE YOUR FAVORITE baking apple, such as Rome, Ida Red, or Honeycrisp. If you're looking for a little variety, use fresh pears in place of the apples.

TOTAL TIME: 40 MINUTES

1. Preheat the oven to 375°F. Cut a thin slice off the rounded end of each apple half to make a flat surface. Pierce around the centers of the apples with a fork about 4 times. Place the apples, cored sides up, in a 9″ baking dish.

2. Sprinkle the apples evenly with the cinnamon and nutmeg. Drizzle with the honey and blend with the spices, using the back of a spoon. Place ¼ cup water in the dish around the apples.

3. Bake for 30 minutes or until tender when pierced with a knife. Sprinkle 1 tablespoon of the granola on each apple and bake for 5 minutes or until heated through. Serve with cooking juices, cheese, and sausages.

MAKES 2 SERVINGS

PER SERVING: 386 calories; 12 g total fat; 7 g saturated fat; 46 g carbohydrate; 7 g fiber; 27 g protein; 61 mg cholesterol; 408 mg sodium

NOTE: To microwave, cover the dish with a sheet of waxed paper and microwave on high for 4 to 5 minutes or until the apples are tender when pierced with a knife. Let stand 5 minutes before serving and top with the granola.

2 large apples (1 pound), halved lengthwise and cored

¼ teaspoon ground cinnamon

⅛ teaspoon grated nutmeg

2 teaspoons honey

4 tablespoons homemade (opposite) or low-fat granola

1 chunk (2 ounces) extra-sharp Cheddar cheese, cut in half

6 ounces cooked Turkey Breakfast Sausage (page 62) or soy breakfast sausages

CHAPTER 4 ○ BREAKFASTS

YOGURT AND BERRY PARFAITS

6 ounces firm tofu

1 tablespoon honey

¾ teaspoon vanilla extract

½ teaspoon lemon zest

1½ cups fat-free plain Greek-style yogurt

1 cup sliced strawberries

1 cup blueberries

½ cup homemade (page 70) or low-fat granola

HERE'S A GREAT way to sneak tofu into the family diet. Save precious morning minutes by slicing the strawberries and making the yogurt mixture up to 1 day in advance. If you prefer a sweeter yogurt, add stevia to taste.

TOTAL TIME: 20 MINUTES

1. Place the tofu, honey, vanilla, and lemon zest in a food processor or blender. Process until smooth. Add the yogurt and pulse until just combined.

2. Spoon ½ cup of the yogurt mixture into each of 2 large parfait glasses or bowls. Top each with ½ cup fruit and 2 tablespoons granola. Repeat layering with the remaining ingredients. Serve immediately.

MAKES 2 SERVINGS

PER SERVING: 412 calories; 9 g total fat; 1 g saturated fat; 56 g carbohydrate; 7 g fiber; 31 g protein; 0 mg cholesterol; 136 mg sodium

---

DIET DILEMMA: ALL-OR-NOTHING ATTITUDE

Problem: What do you do after you start a new diet plan and you slip up? Do you resolve to do better, take a walk, and start right back on the plan with your next meal? Or do you declare yourself a failure and call it quits? If it's the latter, you have an all-or-nothing attitude. You think you're only being successful if you're following a diet to the letter, and any small mistake is grounds for throwing the plan out the window.

Solution: The truth is, everyone is going to make a not-so-great choice every once in a while. You're going to have that second piece of cake at a birthday party or do a bit more damage at the buffet table than you planned. When this happens, don't beat yourself up—just work out a little harder the next day, and start right back with the plan.

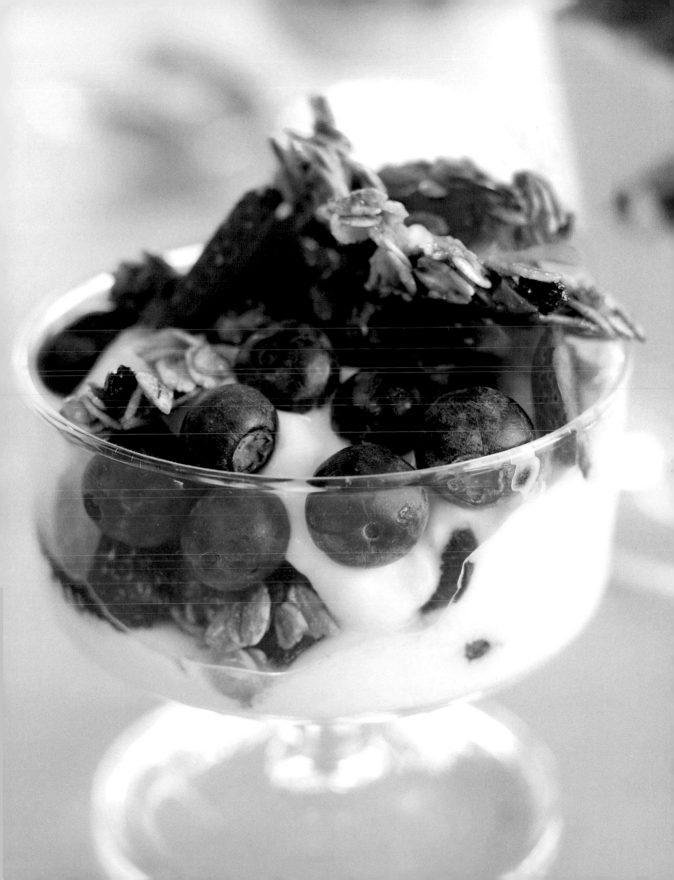

APPLE-BLUEBERRY STEEL-CUT OATS

6 cups fat-free milk, divided

1½ cups steel-cut oats

½ cup dried blueberries

1 large apple, cored and coarsely chopped

¼ teaspoon salt

3 tablespoons honey

1 tablespoon ground flaxseed

¼ teaspoon ground cinnamon

¼ teaspoon apple pie spice

18 ounces prepared Turkey Breakfast Sausage (page 62) or soy breakfast sausage patties

I F YOU LIKE, replace the dried blueberries with an equal amount of dried cherries, golden raisins, or dried cranberries. Great to have on hand, steel-cut oats can be prepared up to 5 days in advance. Single portions can be reheated in the microwave, or in a small saucepan, adding 1 to 2 tablespoons of water for the desired consistency.

TOTAL TIME: 40 MINUTES

1. Bring 1½ cups milk and 2½ cups water just to boiling in a medium saucepan. Stir in the oats, blueberries, apple, and salt. Return to a boil and reduce the heat to low.

2. Cover and simmer, stirring occasionally, for 25 to 30 minutes or until cooked through but still slightly chewy. Stir in the honey, flaxseed, cinnamon, and pie spice. For one portion, serve ¾ cup oatmeal with ¾ cup fat-free milk and 3 ounces sausage.

MAKES 6 SERVINGS

PER SERVING: 351 calories; 3 g total fat; 0 g saturated fat; 52 g carbohydrate; 5 g fiber; 31 g protein; 36 mg cholesterol; 410 mg sodium

---

METABOLISM BOOSTER: FILL UP ON GRAPEFRUIT

While the jury is still out on whether eating grapefruit can speed up metabolism, adding this vitamin C–packed fruit to your diet *can* help with weight loss. One study showed that obese people who ate half a fresh grapefruit before a meal lost significantly more weight than people who didn't eat grapefruit.[3] One theory is that grapefruit eaters filled up on the fruit and so they ate less during their meals. Others speculate that there's a link between grapefruit and insulin; the fruit may reduce levels of this hormone, thereby encouraging weight loss. Regardless of the reason, it's time to become a grapefruit fan, if you aren't one already!

CREAMY BARLEY WITH BERRIES

IRED OF OATMEAL? Here's a fiber-rich hot cereal that's sure to become a favorite. Cooking barley in milk while stirring frequently creates a rich, creamy cereal. This recipe can easily be doubled or tripled.

TOTAL TIME: 15 MINUTES

1. Combine the milk, barley, salt, and cardamom in a small saucepan. Bring to a simmer over medium heat. Cook, stirring frequently, for 15 minutes or until the barley is tender and creamy.

2. Place in a small bowl and drizzle with the honey. Sprinkle with the strawberries and almonds. Serve with the Canadian bacon.

MAKES 1 SERVING

PER SERVING: 403 calories; 8 g total fat; 1 g saturated fat; 62 g carbohydrate; 8 g fiber; 25 g protein; 31 mg cholesterol; 708 mg sodium

NOTE: This recipe is a little high in sodium (you want to aim for no more than 600 to 650 milligrams per meal), so be sure to work this recipe into your daily total of 2,300 milligrams of sodium by selecting recipes for the remaining meals that are around 300 to 400 milligrams each.

1 cup fat-free milk

¼ cup quick-cooking barley

Pinch salt

Pinch cardamom

1 teaspoon honey

1 cup sliced strawberries

1½ tablespoons sliced almonds

2 ounces Canadian bacon or chicken and apple sausage, heated

no-bother breakfasts

10 quick and easy breakfast recipes

breakfast is often referred to as the most important meal of the day. After you've gone 12 or more hours without eating, having a good balanced breakfast is key to successful weight loss and the foundation for sticking with any eating plan. You'll not only prevent hunger, but you'll have the energy to go about your day. Habits such as grabbing a doughnut or bagel are easily dropped when simple, nutritious, and delicious meals are available. Following are 10 such recipes, each ready in as few as 5 and no longer than 15 minutes. For days when time is of the essence, these recipes are sure winners.

The 2-Week Turnaround breakfast should include 400 calories eaten as 2 grains/starchy veggies, 1 dairy, 1 protein, 1 fruit, and 1 fat. Here are some tips used throughout this chapter to be sure your breakfasts provide all the nutrition and energy needed to stick with the exercise and eating plan.

INCLUDE EGG WHITES. Whether you crack them yourself or buy them in a package, egg whites are a great form of protein and perfect for scrambles, omelets, or frittatas. When preparing a favorite dish, substitute two egg whites for each whole egg. Reach for pasteurized egg whites to add to smoothies to pump up the protein.

TOFU TO THE RESCUE. Another way to get protein into your breakfasts is with tofu. Adding soft silken tofu to smoothies or even grain dishes, such as oatmeal and cream of wheat, is a great way to sneak in this important nutrient. Pureed tofu is best for this use and easy to make. Simply place the tofu in a blender or food processor (a mini processor works well for small amounts) and puree just until smooth. If you'd like, puree more than needed for one meal and store in an airtight container in the fridge for up to 3 days.

NUTRITIOUS NUTS. Considered a fat on this plan, 2 tablespoons of nuts helps keep you feeling full while providing a great source of monounsaturated fatty acids (see more about MUFAs on page 18) and protein. Chopped walnuts, pecans, and almonds add crunch and flavor to hot and cold cereals as well as a fun topping on waffles and pancakes. Or stir them into the batter for a hidden treat. Don't forget nut butters like almond or peanut. Delicious spread on toast, nut butters are also delicious as a dip or spread on fruit, especially apples or bananas.

OATMEAL WITH WALNUTS AND PEARS

½ cup old-fashioned oats

3 ounces soft tofu, pureed

1 small pear, finely chopped

1 tablespoon chopped walnuts

⅛ teaspoon vanilla extract

1 cup fat-free milk

1. Cook the oats according to package directions. Stir in the tofu, pear, walnuts, and vanilla. Cook for 1 minute or until heated through.

2. Serve with the milk.

MAKES 1 SERVING

PER SERVING: 423 calories; 9 g total fat; 2 g saturated fat; 66 g carbohydrate; 9 g fiber; 22 g protein; 3 mg cholesterol; 136 mg sodium

BROWN RICE PUDDING

⅔ cup cooked brown rice

3 ounces silken tofu, pureed

1 apple, cored, peeled, and shredded

1 cup fat-free milk

¼ teaspoon ground ginger

2 teaspoons chopped pecans

1½ teaspoon agave nectar

Pinch of salt

1. Combine the rice, tofu, apple, milk, and ginger in a small saucepan and cook, stirring, for 10 minutes or until heated through.

2. Stir in the nectar, pecans, and salt.

MAKES 1 SERVING

PER SERVING: 424 calories; 7 g total fat; 1 g saturated fat; 75 g carbohydrate; 7 g fiber; 17 g protein; 3 mg cholesterol; 142 mg sodium

nutrition notes

● *OATS are packed with fiber, manganese, selenium, and magnesium. and studies show that a diet high in beta-glucan from oats helps to lower blood LDL cholesterol (the bad-for-you cholesterol).*

● *PECANS have been shown to lower cholesterol in clinical studies. They're also higher in antioxidants than any other nut. meaning they may help prevent cell damage that leads to heart disease, Alzheimer's disease. and cancer.*

CHAPTER 4 ○ BREAKFASTS

FARINA WITH PUMPKIN SEEDS

1 cup fat-free milk	2 tablespoons golden raisins
Pinch of salt	1 tablespoon pumpkin seeds
3 tablespoons whole grain farina	1½ teaspoons agave nectar or honey
3 ounces soft tofu, pureed	

Bring the milk, salt, and ¼ cup of water to a boil. Whisk in the farina until smooth. Add the tofu and raisins. Cook according to package directions. Stir in the pumpkin seeds and nectar or honey.

MAKES 1 SERVING

PER SERVING: 386 calories; 8 g total fat; 1 g saturated fat; 61 g carbohydrate; 5 g fiber; 20 g protein; 3 mg cholesterol; 142 mg sodium

CARDAMOM QUINOA PUDDING

½ cup cooked quinoa	Pinch of salt
1 cup fat-free milk, divided	1 teaspoon pine nuts
¼ cup golden raisins	3 ounces vegetarian sausage, cooked
Pinch of ground cardamom	

1. Combine the quinoa, ½ cup milk, raisins, cardamom, and salt in a microwaveable bowl. Microwave on medium, stirring once, for 2 minutes or until heated through. Stir in the pine nuts.

2. Serve the quinoa with the sausage and ½ cup milk.

MAKES 1 SERVING

PER SERVING: 391 calories; 4 g total fat; 0 g saturated fat; 61 g carbohydrate; 5 g fiber; 28 g protein; 3 mg cholesterol; 577 mg sodium

SWISS MUESLI

1 cup fat-free plain Greek-style yogurt

3 ounces soft tofu, pureed

¾ cup whole grain flakes cereal

6 almonds, chopped

1 kiwifruit, chopped

Stir together the yogurt and tofu until well blended in a small bowl. Stir in the cereal, almonds, and kiwi.

MAKES 1 SERVING

PER SERVING: 379 calories; 7 g total fat; 1 g saturated fat; 53 g carbohydrate; 7 g fiber; 30 g protein; 0 mg cholesterol; 201 mg sodium

STUFFED PEACH

½ cup fat-free ricotta cheese

1 teaspoon agave nectar or honey

Pinch of cinnamon

1 small peach or pear, cut in half and pitted or cored

1 serving Turkey Breakfast Sausage (page 62), cooked

½ whole grain English muffin, toasted

2 teaspoons almond butter

1. Stir together the ricotta, nectar or honey, and cinnamon in a small bowl. Place the peach halves on a plate and divide the ricotta mixture onto the halves.

2. Serve with the sausage and the English muffin spread with almond butter.

MAKES 1 SERVING

PER SERVING: 423 calories; 9 g total fat; 1 g saturated fat; 42 g carbohydrate; 4 g fiber; 49 g protein; 55 mg cholesterol; 591 mg sodium

nutrition notes

● A RECENT STUDY *showed that people who ate 3 servings of yogurt per day with a low-calorie diet lost 22 percent more weight and 61 percent more body fat than people who just cut calories.*

● WHOLE GRAINS *are great sources of B vitamins, vitamin E, magnesium, and iron. They also contain lots of fiber to keep you fuller longer—which can help you lose weight.*

WHOLE GRAIN WAFFLE

1 frozen whole grain low-fat waffle

3 ounces vegetarian sausage

2 teaspoons maple syrup

1 cup blueberries

1 cup fat-free milk

1. Prepare the waffle and the sausage according to package directions.
2. Place the waffle on a plate, drizzle with syrup, and sprinkle with the blueberries. Serve with the sausage and milk.

MAKES 1 SERVING

PER SERVING: 397 calories; 4 g total fat; 2 g saturated fat; 68 g carbohydrate; 7 g fiber; 25 g protein; 12 mg cholesterol; 545 mg sodium

WHOLE GRAIN CEREAL AND BANANA

¾ cup whole grain flakes cereal

1 small banana, sliced

2 teaspoons chopped walnuts

1 cup fat-free milk

3 ounces cooked Turkey Breakfast Sausage (page 62)

Combine the cereal, banana, walnuts, and milk in a bowl. Serve with the sausage.

MAKES 1 SERVING

PER SERVING: 407 calories; 3 g total fat; 0 g saturated fat; 61 g carbohydrate; 9 g fiber; 42 g protein; 48 mg cholesterol; 566 mg sodium

CHERRY VANILLA SMOOTHIE

1 multigrain English muffin

2 tablespoons reduced-fat
cream cheese

1 cup unsweetened frozen cherries

1 cup fat-free milk

3 ounces firm silken low-fat tofu

2 teaspoons honey

½ teaspoon vanilla extract

1. Toast the English muffin and spread with cream cheese.

2. Combine the cherries, milk, tofu, honey, and vanilla in a blender and process until smooth. Serve with the English muffin.

MAKES 1 SERVING

PER SERVING: 404 calories; 7 g total fat; 3 g saturated fat; 66 g carbohydrate; 5 g fiber; 22 g protein; 20 mg cholesterol; 377 mg sodium

BANANA SMOOTHIE

1 tablespoon plus 1 teaspoon
soy nut butter

1 small whole wheat pita bread
(4" diameter)

1 small frozen banana

1 cup fat-free milk

3 ounces soft silken tofu

2 teaspoons honey

1. Spread the soy nut butter on the pita bread.

2. Combine the banana, milk, tofu, and honey in a blender and process until smooth. Serve with the pita.

MAKES 1 SERVING

PER SERVING: 397 calories; 7 g total fat; 1 g saturated fat; 68 g carbohydrate; 5 g fiber; 18 g protein; 3 mg cholesterol; 445 mg sodium

nutrition notes

● CHERRIES *are stone fruits, related to plums, peaches, and nectarines. Studies indicate that eating antioxidant-rich cherries may help reduce the risk of many diseases associated with age. including arthritis. heart disease. diabetes. and certain kinds of cancer.*

● BANANAS *are high in potassium. which is essential for maintaining normal blood pressure and heart function.*

LUNCHES

CHAPTER 5 ∘ LUNCHES

"HELP PEOPLE
BECOME MORE
MOTIVATED BY
GUIDING THEM
TO THE SOURCE
OF THEIR OWN
POWER."

—PAUL G. THOMAS

TURKEY CHILI SOUP

12 corn tortillas (6" diameter), cut into 8 wedges

2 tablespoons olive oil

1 onion, chopped

1 small jalapeño chile pepper, seeded and finely chopped (See Note)

2 medium zucchini, chopped

2 teaspoons ground cumin

½ teaspoon chili powder

1 pound 99% fat-free ground turkey breast

1 package (32 ounces) reduced-sodium chicken broth

1 can (15 ounces) kidney beans, rinsed and drained

2 tomatoes, seeded and chopped

½ cup chopped cilantro

THE EASIEST WAY to seed a tomato is to cut it in half crosswise. Using a small spoon, remove and discard the seeds. Then chop or slice as needed. Store any leftover soup in an airtight container in the refrigerator for up to 3 days or freeze for up to 2 months. Store the tortilla crisps in a resealable bag for up to 3 days.

TOTAL TIME: 50 MINUTES

1. Preheat the oven to 400°F. Coat 2 baking sheets with cooking spray. Add the tortillas in a single layer and spray with cooking spray. Bake for 5 to 8 minutes or until crisp. Set aside.

2. Heat the oil in a large saucepan over medium-high heat. Add the onion and chile pepper; cook, stirring occasionally, for 5 minutes or until lightly browned. Stir in the zucchini, cumin, and chili powder. Cook for 10 minutes or until the zucchini is lightly browned.

3. Add the turkey and cook, stirring to break up with a spoon, for 5 minutes or until no longer pink. Stir in the broth, beans, and tomatoes. Bring to a boil over high heat. Reduce the heat to low and simmer for 15 minutes.

4. Remove from the heat. Stir in the cilantro.

MAKES 6 SERVINGS

PER SERVING: 321 calories; 8 g total fat; 1 g saturated fat; 37 g carbohydrate; 8 g fiber; 29 g protein; 33 mg cholesterol; 383 mg sodium

NOTE: Wear plastic gloves and keep hands away from eyes when handling fresh chile peppers.

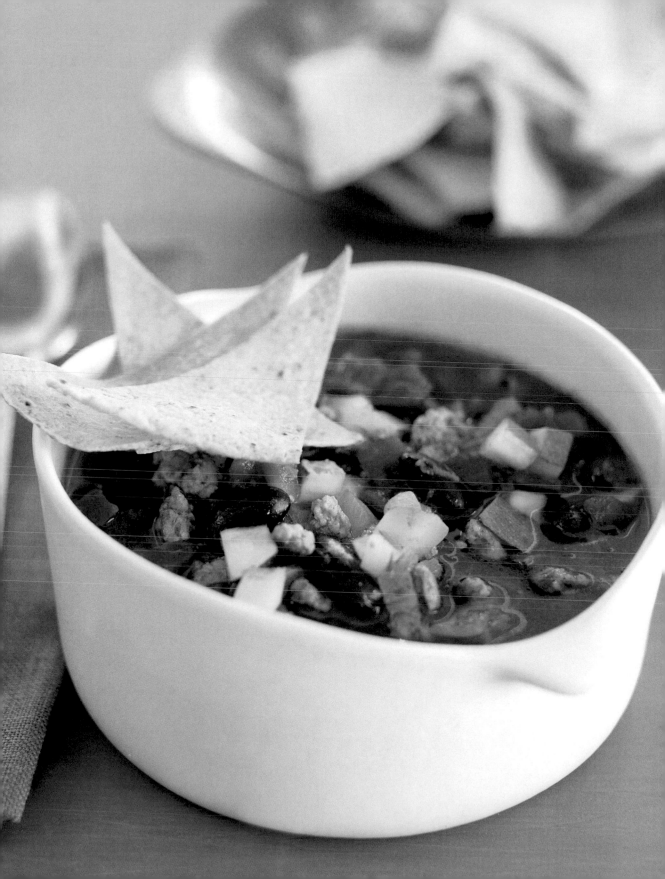

PARSNIP AND APPLE SOUP WITH TURKEY MELT

1 pound parsnips, peeled and chopped

2 large apples, peeled, cored, and chopped

2 ribs celery, chopped

1 onion, chopped

1½ teaspoons ground ginger

¼ teaspoon ground cardamom

1 package (32 ounces) reduced-sodium chicken broth, divided

4 slices thin whole grain bread

4 teaspoons honey mustard

12 ounces low-sodium deli turkey breast

4 thin slices (½ ounce each) reduced-fat Jarlsberg cheese

NOTHING BEATS HOT soup and a sandwich to warm your bones and fill your belly. Here the flavors of autumn are highlighted in a rich soup featuring parsnips, apples, and ginger. For a change of pace, substitute butternut squash for the parsnips.

TOTAL TIME: 40 MINUTES

1. Bring the parsnips, apples, celery, onion, ginger, cardamom, and 3 cups of the broth to a boil in a large saucepan. Reduce the heat to low, cover, and simmer for 25 minutes or until the parsnips are very tender.

2. Meanwhile, preheat the oven to broil. Place the bread on a broiler pan and broil 1 side for 3 minutes or until toasted. Turn, spread with the mustard, and top with the turkey and cheese. Just before serving, place under the broiler to melt the cheese.

3. Transfer the parsnip mixture to a food processor, working in batches if necessary. Puree until smooth. Return to the saucepan and add the remaining 1 cup of broth.

4. Divide the soup among 4 bowls and serve with a turkey melt.

MAKES 4 SERVINGS

PER SERVING: 376 calories; 5 g total fat; 2 g saturated fat; 55 g carbohydrate; 11 g fiber; 35 g protein; 53 mg cholesterol; 415 mg sodium

TUSCAN
SOUP

chris's favorites

" THIS HEARTY SOUP made with turkey sausage is a family favorite! I'm also a big fan of sneaking spinach into any meal I can. Spinach cooks down, has a mild taste, and it's also full of vitamins."

TOTAL TIME: 25 MINUTES

1. Heat the oil in a large saucepot or Dutch oven over medium heat. Cook the sausage, stirring occasionally, for 5 minutes or until browned.

2. Add the onion and cook for 3 minutes or until translucent. Add the zucchini and garlic and cook for 3 minutes or until tender.

3. Add the oregano, tomatoes with their juice, broth, and beans. Bring to a boil and cook for 2 minutes. Reduce the heat to low, add the spinach and cheese, and cook for 2 minutes or until wilted.

MAKES 4 SERVINGS

PER SERVING: 336 calories; 14 g total fat; 4 g saturated fat; 22 g carbohydrate; 6 g fiber; 29 g protein; 60 mg cholesterol; 891 mg sodium

NOTE: This recipe is a little high in sodium (you want to aim for no more than 600 to 650 milligrams per meal), so be sure to work this recipe into your daily total of 2,300 milligrams of sodium by selecting recipes for the remaining meals that are around 300 to 400 milligrams each.

2 tablespoons olive oil

12 ounces low-fat turkey sausage, sliced

1 small onion, chopped

1 medium zucchini, chopped

1 clove garlic, minced

½ teaspoon dried oregano

1 can (14.5 ounces) no-salt-added diced tomatoes

1 package (32 ounces) reduced-sodium chicken broth

1 can (19 ounces) cannellini beans, rinsed and drained

4 cups chopped spinach

¼ cup grated Parmesan cheese

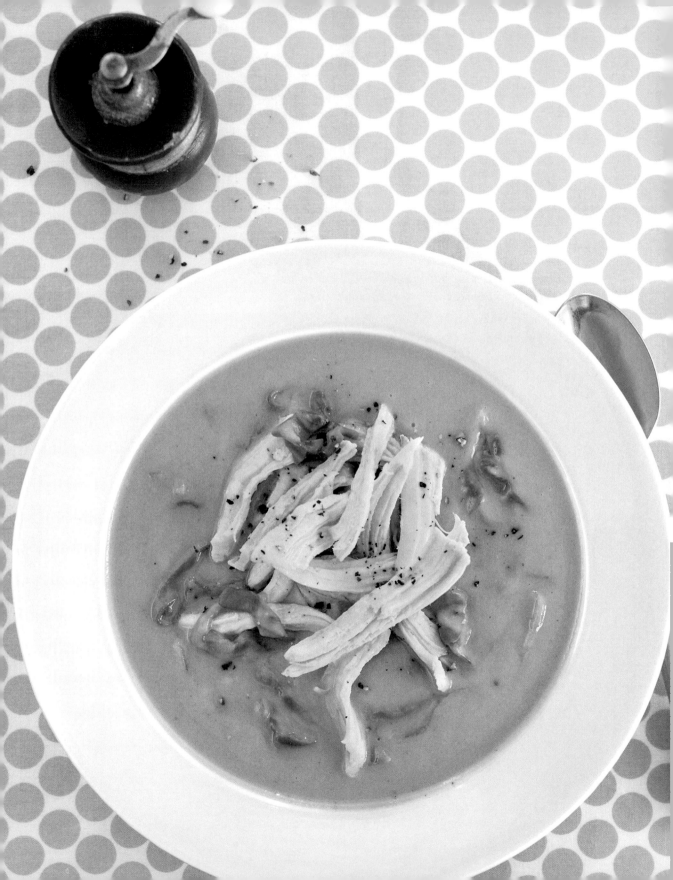

SPICY SWEET POTATO SOUP WITH CHICKEN

S AVE TIME IN the kitchen by substituting 2½ cups baby carrots for the whole carrots in this recipe. To add a bit of spicy zest to the soup, stir in some red or green hot-pepper sauce.

TOTAL TIME: 45 MINUTES

1. Heat the oil in a large saucepan over medium-high heat. Cook the onion for 5 minutes, stirring occasionally, until lightly browned. Stir in the garlic, curry powder, and ginger. Cook for 1 minute or until fragrant.

2. Stir in the carrots, sweet potatoes, and 3 cups of the broth. Bring to a boil, reduce the heat to low, cover, and simmer for 20 minutes or until the carrots and sweet potatoes are tender.

3. Transfer to a food processor, working in batches if necessary. Puree the hot mixture until smooth. Return to the saucepan and add the spinach and the remaining 1 cup of broth. Bring to a simmer.

4. Remove from the heat. Divide among 4 bowls and top with the chicken. Sprinkle with freshly ground pepper to taste.

MAKES 4 SERVINGS

PER SERVING: 368 calories; 11 g total fat; 2 g saturated fat; 37 g carbohydrate; 9 g fiber; 30 g protein; 68 mg cholesterol; 335 mg sodium

2 tablespoons olive oil

1 large onion, chopped

2 cloves garlic, minced

2 teaspoons ground curry powder

1 teaspoon ground ginger

4 carrots, sliced

1 pound sweet potatoes, peeled and cut into 1" chunks

1 package (32 ounces) reduced-sodium chicken broth, divided

12 ounces cooked chicken breast, shredded (about 3 cups)

1 package (7 to 9 ounces) baby spinach

CREAM OF BROCCOLI SOUP

2 tablespoons olive oil, divided

1 large onion, chopped

1 yellow bell pepper, chopped

1 clove garlic, minced

2 cups reduced-sodium vegetable or chicken broth, divided

1 large bunch (1 pound) broccoli, stem and florets coarsely chopped

2 russet potatoes, peeled and chopped

12 ounces Canadian bacon, diced

ADDING POTATO TO the soup creates a rich creaminess without the added fat and calories of heavy cream. The yellow bell peppers add a nice flavor to traditional broccoli soup.

TOTAL TIME: 55 MINUTES

1. Heat 1 tablespoon of the oil in a large saucepot over medium heat. Cook the onion and pepper for 5 minutes or until lightly browned. Add the garlic and cook for 1 minute. Add 1 cup of the broth, the broccoli, potatoes, and 2 cups water. Bring to a boil, reduce the heat to low, cover, and simmer for 30 minutes or until the broccoli stems and potatoes are very tender.

2. Meanwhile, heat the remaining 1 tablespoon of oil in a medium skillet over medium-high heat. Cook the bacon, stirring constantly, for 5 minutes or until browned and crisp. Set aside.

3. Transfer the soup to a food processor, working in batches if necessary. Puree the hot mixture until smooth. Return to the pot and add the remaining 1 cup of broth. Stir in the bacon.

MAKES 4 SERVINGS

PER SERVING: 344 calories; 12 g total fat; 3 g saturated fat; 39 g carbohydrate; 5 g fiber; 21 g protein; 31 mg cholesterol; 897 mg sodium

NOTE: This recipe is a little high in sodium (you want to aim for no more than 600 to 650 milligrams per meal), so be sure to work this recipe into your daily total of 2,300 milligrams of sodium by selecting recipes for the remaining meals that are around 300 to 400 milligrams each.

AVOCADO SOUP WITH SPICY SHRIMP

THE QUICKEST WAY to ripen avocados is in a paper bag, preferably with an apple. Avocados yield to gentle pressure when ripe. Removing the stem can also determine ripeness: If the stem comes off easily and the flesh is green, it's ripe. If the stem holds on it's not quite ripe, so wait another day and test again.

TOTAL TIME: 25 MINUTES

1. Combine the shrimp and seasoning in a shallow bowl, tossing to coat well. Set aside.

2. Preheat the oven to 400°F. Coat a baking sheet with cooking spray. Add the tortillas in a single layer and spray with cooking spray. Bake for 5 minutes or until crisp. Set aside.

3. Place the scallions, avocados, buttermilk, cilantro, garlic, lime juice, and salt in a blender and puree until smooth. Set aside.

4. Heat a large skillet coated with cooking spray over medium-high heat. Add the shrimp and cook, stirring, for 5 to 7 minutes or until the shrimp are opaque.

5. Divide the soup among 4 bowls. Top with the shrimp and serve with the chips.

MAKES 4 SERVINGS

PER SERVING: 425 calories; 19 g total fat; 3 g saturated fat; 39 g carbohydrate; 10 g fiber; 28 g protein; 173 mg cholesterol; 554 mg sodium

1 pound large shrimp, peeled and deveined

1 tablespoon Cajun seasoning

4 corn tortillas (6" diameter), cut into 1" strips

4 scallions, coarsely chopped

2 avocados, halved, pitted, and peeled

2 cups reduced-fat buttermilk

1 cup chopped cilantro

1 clove garlic

3 tablespoons fresh lime juice

¼ teaspoon salt

VEGETABLE FISH SOUP WITH ROUILLE

1 large onion, cut into wedges

1 package (32 ounces) reduced-sodium vegetable broth

2 tablespoons frozen orange juice concentrate

4 small red potatoes, washed and quartered (about 1 pound)

1 package (9 ounces) frozen artichoke hearts, thawed

1 pound firm fish such as cod, scrod, pollock, snapper, or turbot, cut into 1½" pieces

¾ cup Swiss chard, cut into 1" pieces

2 roasted red peppers, drained and patted dry

1 clove garlic

½ teaspoon Dijon mustard

2 tablespoons olive oil

¼ teaspoon hot-pepper sauce

A ROUILLE IS A spicy red-pepper sauce often made of hot red chiles. Here a milder version is prepared with roasted red peppers and a touch of spice from hot-pepper sauce.

TOTAL TIME: 40 MINUTES

1. Heat a large saucepot coated with cooking spray over medium-high heat. Cook the onion, stirring, for 5 minutes or until lightly browned. Add the broth, orange juice concentrate, and potatoes. Bring to a boil. Reduce the heat to low, cover, and simmer for 20 minutes or until the potatoes are almost fork-tender.

2. Stir in the artichoke hearts and fish. Return to a simmer and cook for 4 minutes or until the potatoes are tender and the fish is opaque. Stir in the chard during the last 2 minutes of cooking.

3. Meanwhile, to make the rouille, combine the peppers, garlic, and mustard in a food processor or blender and puree. Gradually pour in the oil and hot-pepper sauce with the processor running. Divide the soup among 4 bowls. Top each with one-quarter of the rouille.

MAKES 4 SERVINGS

PER SERVING: 319 calories; 8 g total fat; 1 g saturated fat; 37 g carbohydrate; 8 g fiber; 25 g protein; 49 mg cholesterol; 684 mg sodium

NOTE: This recipe is a little high in sodium (you want to aim for no more than 600 to 650 milligrams per meal), so be sure to work this recipe into your daily total of 2,300 milligrams of sodium by selecting recipes for the remaining meals that are around 300 to 400 milligrams each.

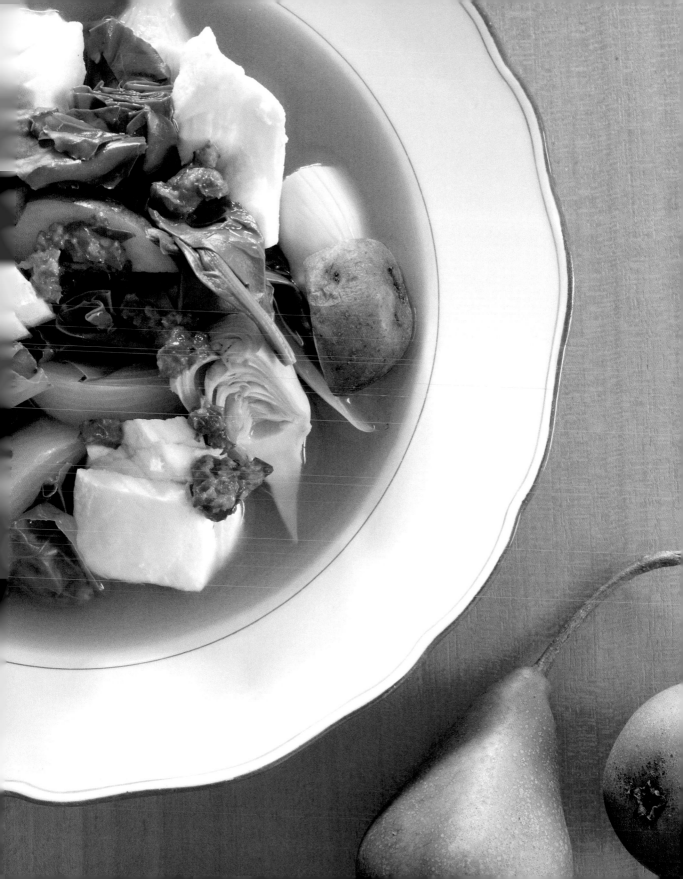

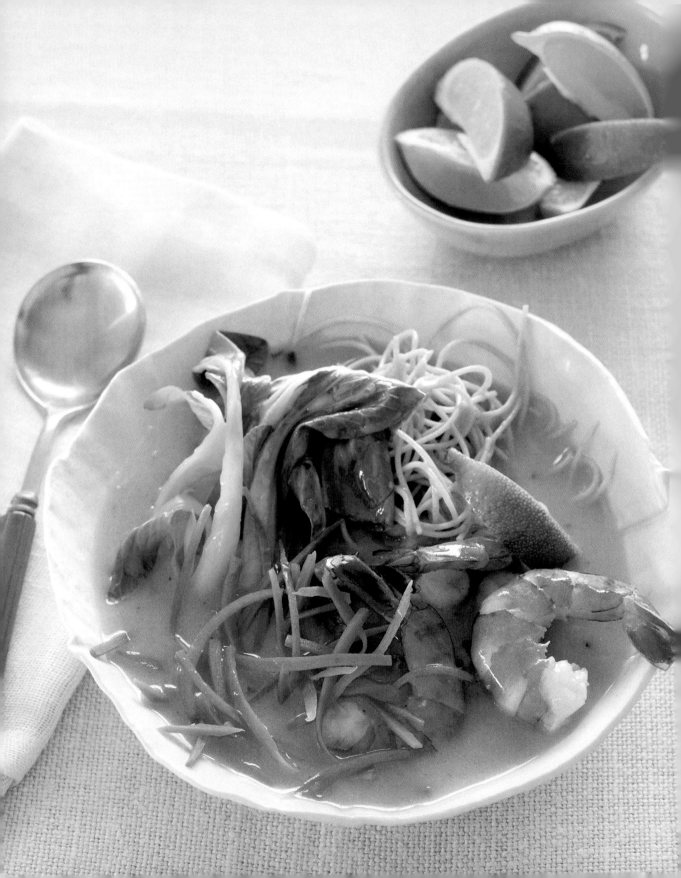

COCONUT-LIME SHRIMP SOUP

THIS COLORFUL, TASTY soup features classic Thai flavors, especially creamy coconut milk. Look for coconut milk in the international section of your supermarket. Always choose the light variety, which has less than half the fat and calories of regular coconut milk.

TOTAL TIME: 30 MINUTES

1. Coat a large saucepan with cooking spray. Add the carrots, bok choy, garlic, and ginger and cook, stirring, for 3 minutes or until fragrant. Add the broth, coconut milk, soy sauce, curry paste, and 1 cup of water. Cook just until the mixture comes to a boil over medium-high heat.

2. Add the pasta; return just to a boil. Reduce the heat to medium and simmer for 4 minutes or until almost tender. Stir in the shrimp. Cook for 1 to 3 minutes or until the shrimp are opaque and the pasta is tender. Remove from the heat and stir in the lime juice.

MAKES 4 SERVINGS

PER SERVING: 365 calories; 10 g total fat; 6 g saturated fat; 34 g carbohydrate; 5 g fiber; 34 g protein; 175 mg cholesterol; 495 mg sodium

4 carrots, cut into julienne strips

3 heads baby bok choy, sliced

1 clove garlic, minced

1 tablespoon grated fresh ginger

2 cups reduced-sodium chicken broth

1 can (13.5 to 14 ounces) light coconut milk

2 teaspoons reduced-sodium soy sauce

¼ to ½ teaspoon red or green curry paste

4 ounces multigrain or whole wheat angel hair pasta, broken in half

1 pound large shrimp, peeled and deveined

2 tablespoons lime juice

MUSHROOM BARLEY SOUP WITH SPINACH AND SAUSAGE

1 ounce dried porcini
mushrooms

12 ounces frozen soy
sausages

½ pound sliced cremini
or button mushrooms

2 shallots, finely chopped

2 carrots, chopped

2 ribs celery, chopped

1 cup quick-cooking barley

2 cloves garlic, minced

1 teaspoon dried thyme

1 package (32 ounces)
low-sodium beef or
vegetable broth

1 package (7 to 9 ounces)
baby spinach

T O BENEFIT THE most from the healing properties of garlic, crush or mince it and let it stand for 10 minutes before cooking. This will release the healing compounds, which are usually deactivated if the garlic is cooked immediately after mincing.

TOTAL TIME: 45 MINUTES

1. Soak the dried mushrooms in 1 cup boiling water in a medium bowl for 30 minutes.

2. Meanwhile, cook the sausages in a large saucepot or Dutch oven over medium heat for 8 minutes, turning occasionally until browned. Remove to a plate; chop into bite-size pieces and set aside.

3. Coat the same pot with cooking spray and place over medium-high heat. Cook the cremini mushrooms, shallots, carrots, and celery, stirring occasionally, for 10 minutes or until browned. Add the barley, garlic, and thyme and cook, stirring, for 2 minutes.

4. Remove the reconstituted mushrooms from the liquid, reserving the liquid. Chop the mushrooms and add to the pot. Stir in the broth, reserved liquid, and 2 cups water. Bring to a boil. Reduce the heat to low, cover, and simmer for 10 minutes or until the barley is tender.

5. Stir in the spinach and sausage. Cook for 2 minutes or until the spinach wilts.

MAKES 4 SERVINGS

PER SERVING: 355 calories; 2 g total fat; 1 g saturated fat; 59 g carbohydrate; 11 g fiber; 28 g protein; 0 mg cholesterol; 629 mg sodium

MISO NOODLE BOWL

MISO IS FERMENTED soybean paste that's very common in Japanese cooking. It's sold by color—dark, red, light, and yellow. You'll want to go for the light or yellow varieties, as they are less salty than the darker ones.

TOTAL TIME: 20 MINUTES

1. Prepare the pasta according to package directions. Drain.

2. Meanwhile, bring the broth, ginger, and 3 cups water to a boil in a large saucepot or Dutch oven over high heat. Add the carrots and broccoli and return to boiling. Reduce the heat to low, cover, and simmer for 5 minutes or until the vegetables are tender-crisp.

3. Place the miso in a small bowl and whisk in about 3 tablespoons of the broth mixture until smooth. Pour into the pot. Stir in the pasta, tofu, scallions, and oil and simmer for 3 minutes or until heated through.

MAKES 4 SERVINGS

PER SERVING: 310 calories; 8 g total fat; 1 g saturated fat; 47 g carbohydrate; 10 g fiber; 16 g protein; 0 mg cholesterol; 781 mg sodium

NOTE: This recipe is a little high in sodium (you want to aim for no more than 600 to 650 milligrams per meal), so be sure to work this recipe into your daily total of 2,300 milligrams of sodium by selecting recipes for the remaining meals that are around 300 to 400 milligrams each.

4 ounces whole wheat angel hair pasta

2 cups vegetable or chicken broth

1 teaspoon ground ginger

2 carrots, diagonally sliced

1 head broccoli (about 1 pound), cut into florets

¼ cup miso (any flavor)

16 ounces silken tofu, cut into ¼" cubes

4 scallions, sliced

1 tablespoon toasted sesame oil

SPINACH-STUFFED TOMATO

2 large tomatoes

1 tablespoon olive oil

1 small red onion, chopped

1 clove garlic, minced

½ teaspoon ground coriander

⅛ teaspoon salt

2 drops hot-pepper sauce

6 ounces 99% fat-free ground turkey breast

1 cup cooked brown rice

3 cups baby spinach

¼ cup low-fat crumbled feta cheese

YOU MIGHT FIND it unusual to have a warm filling in a raw tomato, but give it a shot. Bursting with rich flavors, this filling is so delicious it complements the tomato beautifully.

TOTAL TIME: 20 MINUTES

1. Cut the tops off of the tomatoes and scoop out the pulp and seeds. Chop the tops and pulp and place in a sieve over a bowl. Set aside. Place the tomatoes onto 2 plates. If you want a fancier presentation, cut down the sides to fan the tomatoes without cutting through.

2. Heat the oil in a large skillet over medium heat. Cook the onion, stirring, for 3 minutes or until lightly browned. Add the garlic, coriander, salt, and hot-pepper sauce and cook, stirring, for 1 minute.

3. Add the turkey and cook, stirring, for 3 minutes or until no longer pink. Stir in the chopped tomato, rice, and spinach and cook for 3 minutes or until heated through and the spinach wilts.

4. Remove from the heat. Stir in the feta. Stuff the tomatoes with the mixture.

MAKES 2 SERVINGS

PER SERVING: 391 calories; 12 g total fat; 3 g saturated fat; 39 g carbohydrate; 7 g fiber; 37 g protein; 50 mg cholesterol; 591 mg sodium

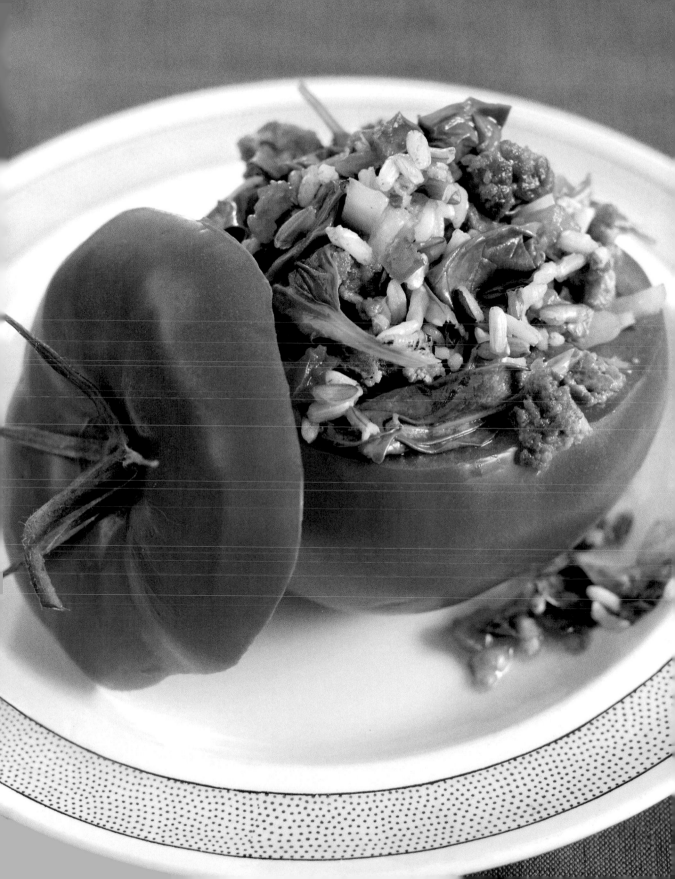

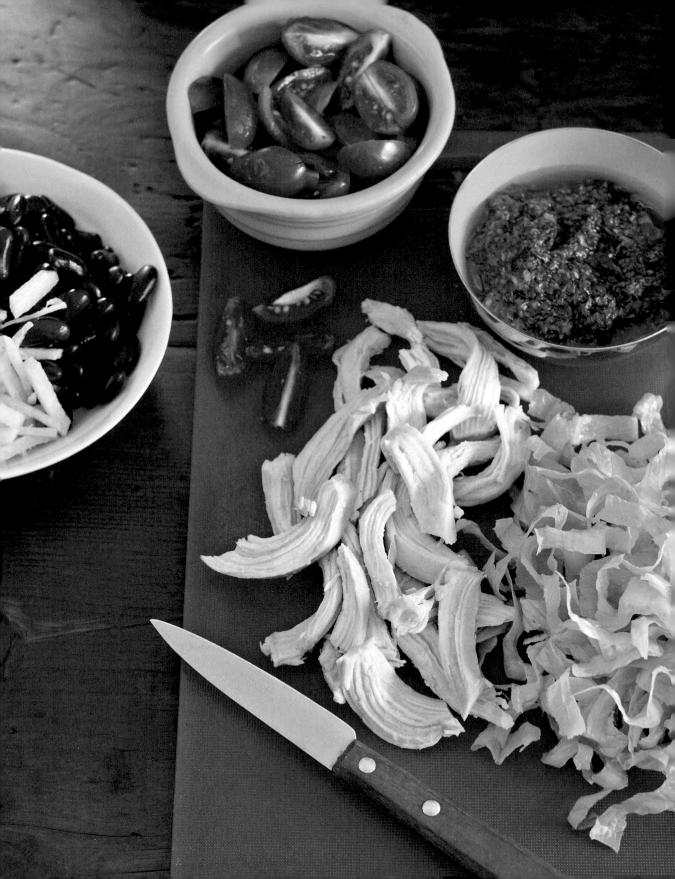

MEXICAN CHOPPED SALAD

THIS RECIPE SERVES 4, but if you'd like to have just 1 or 2 servings, you can prepare the full recipe of the dressing and keep it in the refrigerator for up to 4 days. Then just halve the salad ingredients.

TOTAL TIME: 20 MINUTES

1. Combine the cilantro, garlic, lime juice, cumin, and salt in a food processor or blender. Pulse until chopped. Add the olive oil in a stream, pulsing until emulsified.

2. Arrange the romaine on a serving plate. Place the chicken, beans, jicama, and tomato in piles on the romaine. Drizzle with the dressing.

MAKES 4 SERVINGS

PER SERVING: 386 calories; 18 g total fat; 3 g saturated fat; 26 g carbohydrate; 12 g fiber; 30 g protein; 64 mg cholesterol; 324 mg sodium

½ cup cilantro

1 small clove garlic

2 tablespoons fresh lime juice

½ teaspoon ground cumin

⅛ teaspoon salt

¼ cup olive oil

6 cups chopped romaine lettuce

12 ounces cooked chicken, shredded (about 3 cups)

1 can (15 ounces) pinto or kidney beans, rinsed and drained

1 small jicama (about 8 ounces), peeled and chopped

1 cup grape tomatoes, quartered

PESTO POTATO AND SNAP BEAN SALAD

12 ounces chicken sausage

3 tablespoons prepared pesto

2 tablespoons fat-free plain Greek-style yogurt

2 tablespoons low-fat mayonnaise

4 medium red potatoes, scrubbed and cut into quarters

½ pound green beans, trimmed and cut in half

1 cup cherry tomatoes, halved

2 scallions, sliced

A QUICK WAY TO trim green or snap beans is to gather them into a bunch, lining up the stem ends on a cutting board. Cut off the stem ends with a sharp paring knife.

TOTAL TIME: 20 MINUTES

1. Grill or broil the chicken sausage according to package directions.

2. Meanwhile, stir together the pesto, yogurt, and mayonnaise in a large bowl. Set aside.

3. Bring 2″ of water to a boil in a large saucepan over high heat. Place a steamer basket in the pan and add the potatoes. Cover and cook over medium heat for 15 minutes or until slightly tender. Add the green beans, cover, and cook for 4 minutes or until the potatoes are tender and the beans are tender-crisp. Add to the bowl with the dressing, gently tossing to coat well.

4. Stir in the tomatoes and scallions. Divide the sausages and salad among 4 plates.

MAKES 4 SERVINGS

PER SERVING: 350 calories; 12 g total fat; 3 g saturated fat; 43 g carbohydrate; 5 g fiber; 20 g protein; 64 mg cholesterol; 613 mg sodium

GREEN GODDESS CHICKEN SALAD

THE BEST WAY to cut an avocado in half is to insert a chef's knife through the skin to the pit. Continue cutting all the way around the avocado pit. Twist the halves apart. Insert the knife into the pit and twist the avocado away from the pit.

TOTAL TIME: 20 MINUTES

1. Puree the avocado, yogurt, lemon juice, tarragon, and salt in a blender. Place in a large bowl.

2. Stir in the chicken, radishes, and celery. Toss until well blended.

3. Divide the mixed greens, tomatoes, and cucumber onto 4 plates. Top with the chicken salad. Serve with the crispbreads.

MAKES 4 SERVINGS

PER SERVING: 325 calories; 8 g total fat; 1 g saturated fat; 32 g carbohydrate; 5 g fiber; 32 g protein; 64 mg cholesterol; 268 mg sodium

1 small ripe avocado, halved, pitted, and peeled

¾ cup fat-free plain Greek-style yogurt

1 tablespoon lemon juice

2 tablespoons chopped fresh tarragon

¼ teaspoon salt

12 ounces cooked chicken, shredded (about 3 cups)

8 radishes, chopped

2 ribs celery, chopped

4 cups mixed greens

2 tomatoes, cut into wedges

1 small cucumber, scored and sliced

16 whole grain crispbreads

NOODLE SALAD WITH PEANUT SAUCE

¼ cup natural creamy peanut butter

2 tablespoons rice wine vinegar

1 tablespoon reduced-sodium soy sauce

1 tablespoon toasted sesame oil

1 teaspoon honey

½ teaspoon ground ginger

Pinch red-pepper flakes

4 ounces soba (buckwheat) noodles

2 carrots, cut into julienne strips

6 ounces snow peas, strings removed and cut into thin strips

1 small red bell pepper, cut into julienne strips

12 ounces baked teriyaki or smoked tofu, diced

WHEN PURCHASING SOBA noodles, select ones with the most buckwheat, preferably 100 percent. As you stir the sauce, the peanut butter may look curdled at one point. Don't worry—simply continue whisking and the ingredients will come together to make a creamy sauce.

TOTAL TIME: 25 MINUTES

1. Whisk together the peanut butter, vinegar, soy sauce, sesame oil, honey, ginger, and red-pepper flakes in a large bowl. Set aside.

2. Cook the noodles in a large pot of boiling water over high heat for 2 minutes. Add the carrots, snow peas, and bell pepper. Cook for 3 minutes longer. Drain, reserving ⅓ cup of the water. Rinse the noodles and vegetables under cold water. Drain well.

3. Whisk the reserved water into the peanut mixture until smooth. Add the noodles, carrots, snow peas, bell pepper, and tofu, tossing to coat well.

MAKES 4 SERVINGS

PER SERVING: 452 calories; 21 g total fat; 3 g saturated fat; 39 g carbohydrate; 5 g fiber; 29 g protein; 0 mg cholesterol; 812 mg sodium

NOTE: This recipe is a little high in sodium (you want to aim for no more than 600 to 650 milligrams per meal), so be sure to work this recipe into your daily total of 2,300 milligrams of sodium by selecting recipes for the remaining meals that are around 300 to 400 milligrams each.

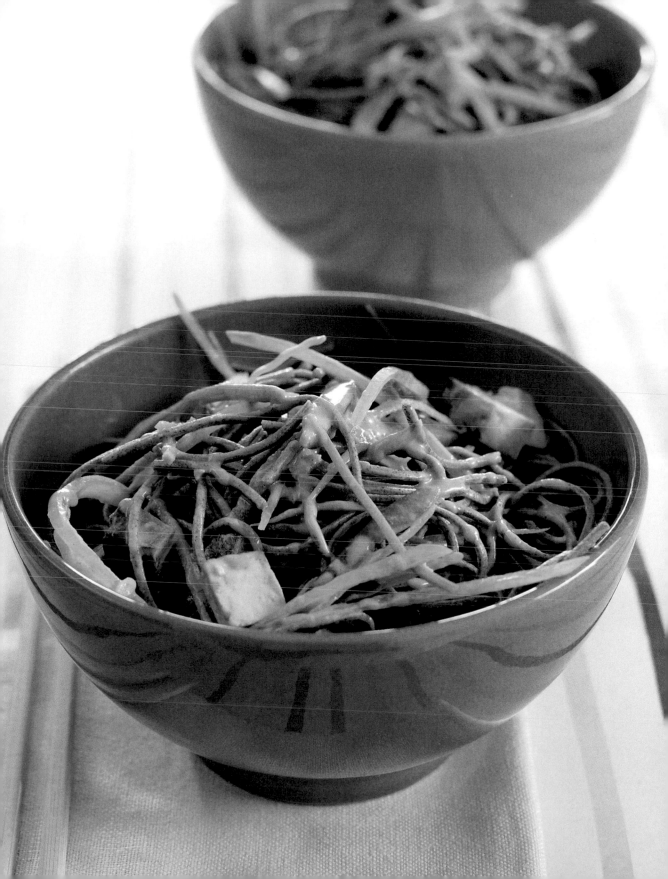

SPINACH SALAD WITH CHICKEN SAUSAGE

4 thick slices (2 ounces each) whole grain bread, cut into 1" cubes

½ teaspoon dried thyme

2 tablespoons olive oil, divided

8 ounces sliced shiitake mushrooms

12 ounces chicken and apple sausage, sliced

2 shallots, finely chopped

2 tablespoons white, balsamic, sherry, or white wine vinegar

⅛ teaspoon salt

⅛ teaspoon pepper

6 cups baby spinach

USE WHOLE GRAIN bread from the bakery for the croutons instead of presliced sandwich bread. Thick, dense slices studded with a variety of whole grains make hearty, delicious croutons.

TOTAL TIME: 20 MINUTES

1. Preheat the oven to 425°F.

2. Place the bread cubes on a baking sheet, coat with cooking spray, and sprinkle with the thyme. Bake for 5 minutes or until browned and crisp.

3. Heat 1 tablespoon of the oil in a large skillet over medium-high heat. Cook the mushrooms for 5 minutes or until browned and tender. Add the sausage and cook for 3 minutes or until the sausage is browned. Remove with a slotted spoon to a plate; set aside.

4. Add the remaining 1 tablespoon of oil to the skillet. Cook the shallots for 3 minutes. Add the vinegar, stirring to break up the brown bits. Remove from the heat. Stir in the salt and pepper.

5. Place the spinach in a large bowl. Toss with the mushroom mixture and drizzle with the vinaigrette. Top with the croutons.

MAKES 4 SERVINGS

PER SERVING: 329 calories; 16 g total fat; 3 g saturated fat; 37 g carbohydrate; 10 g fiber; 18 g protein; 62 mg cholesterol; 708 mg sodium

NOTE: This recipe is a little high in sodium (you want to aim for no more than 600 to 650 milligrams per meal), so be sure to work this recipe into your daily total of 2,300 milligrams of sodium by selecting recipes for the remaining meals that are around 300 to 400 milligrams each.

WARM LENTIL SALAD

CRUSHING DRIED HERBS releases the flavor-carrying essential oils, adding the maximum flavor to recipes. Rub them between the palms of your hands to crush.

TOTAL TIME: 35 MINUTES

1. Bring the lentils and 4 cups of water to a boil in a medium saucepan over high heat. Reduce the heat to low, cover, and simmer for 15 minutes or until tender.

2. Whisk together the vinegar, honey, and mustard until blended. Whisk in 2 tablespoons of the oil. Set aside.

3. Heat the remaining 1 tablespoon of oil in a large skillet over medium-high heat. Cook the bacon for 5 minutes, stirring constantly, until browned. Remove with a slotted spoon to a bowl.

4. Add the carrots, celery, onion, and thyme and cook, stirring, for 8 minutes or until browned and tender. Add to the bowl with the vinaigrette. Stir in the bacon and the drained lentils. Toss to coat well.

5. Place the frisée on a large plate. Top with the lentil mixture and sprinkle with the cheese.

MAKES 4 SERVINGS

PER SERVING: 359 calories; 16 g total fat; 3 g saturated fat; 37 g carbohydrate; 9 g fiber; 20 g protein; 23 mg cholesterol; 812 mg sodium

NOTE: This recipe is a little high in sodium (you want to aim for no more than 600 to 650 milligrams per meal), so be sure to work this recipe into your daily total of 2,300 milligrams of sodium by selecting recipes for the remaining meals that are around 300 to 400 milligrams each.

¾ cup green lentils

2 tablespoons white wine vinegar

1 tablespoon honey

1 tablespoon Dijon mustard

3 tablespoons olive oil, divided

8 ounces Canadian bacon, chopped

2 carrots, chopped

2 ribs celery, chopped

1 red onion, chopped

1 teaspoon dried thyme

6 cups frisée or mixed greens, torn into bite-size pieces

2 ounces low-fat goat cheese

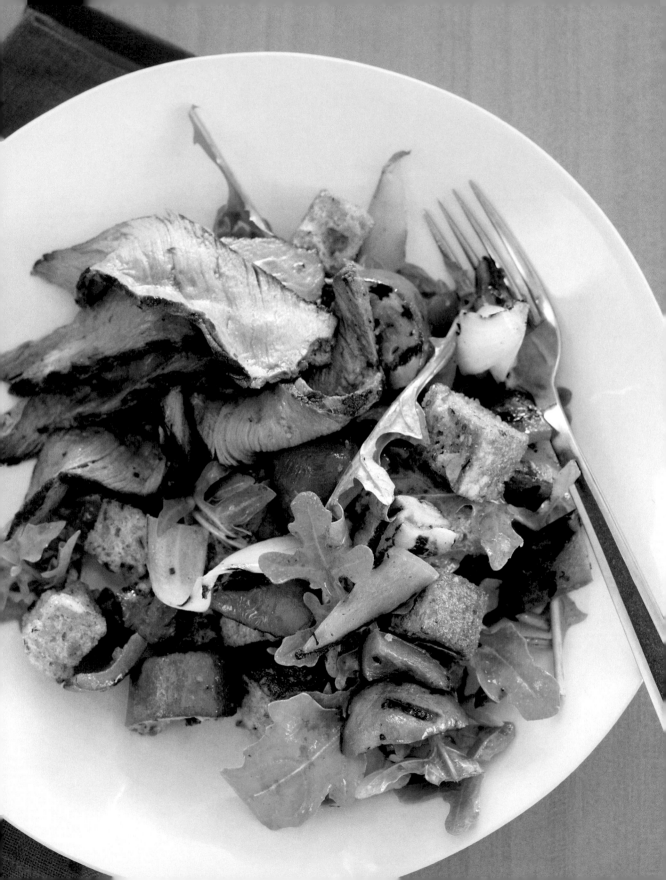

GRILLED PANZANELLA SALAD

THIS SALAD IS the perfect accompaniment to leftover meats and fish. Skip step 3, and replace the steak with 12 ounces of leftover chicken, beef, or fish.

TOTAL TIME: 50 MINUTES

1. Coat a vegetable grill rack or broiler pan with cooking spray. Preheat the grill or broiler. Place the eggplant, zucchini, bell pepper, and onion on the rack or pan. Coat with cooking spray. Sprinkle the steak with the salt and pepper.

2. Grill or broil the vegetables, turning occasionally, for 15 minutes or until browned and tender.

3. Grill or broil the steak, turning once, for 8 minutes or until a thermometer inserted in the center registers 145°F for medium-rare, 160°F for medium, or 165°F for well-done. Let stand for 10 minutes before slicing.

4. Coat the bread with cooking spray and add to the pan used for the vegetables. Grill or broil, turning once, for 2 to 3 minutes or until browned. Place the vegetables and bread in a large bowl.

5. Add the basil, arugula, and vinaigrette to the bowl with the bread and vegetables; toss to coat well. Slice the steak.

6. Divide the steak and salad among 4 plates and serve immediately.

MAKES 4 SERVINGS

PER SERVING: 326 calories; 8 g total fat; 2 g saturated fat; 40 g carbohydrate; 8 g fiber; 28 g protein; 40 mg cholesterol; 363 mg sodium

1 small (8 ounces) eggplant, peeled and cut into 1" pieces

1 zucchini, cut into 1" pieces

1 red bell pepper, cut into 1" pieces

1 onion, cut into thin wedges

12 ounces top round sirloin steak

¼ teaspoon salt

¼ teaspoon pepper

4 thick slices (2 ounces each) 9-grain bread, cut into 1" cubes

1 cup basil leaves

6 cups baby arugula

⅓ cup bottled low-fat balsamic vinaigrette

TEX-MEX TUNA AND BEAN SALAD

3 tablespoons lime juice

1 tablespoon chopped fresh cilantro

1 teaspoon lime zest

3 tablespoons olive oil

1 can (6 ounces) tuna packed in water, drained

1 cup black beans, rinsed and drained

1 roasted red pepper, chopped

½ small red onion, cut into thin strips

4 cups baby romaine lettuce

BE SURE TO rinse canned beans well before using to remove up to 40 percent of the sodium added to the can. This recipe can be adapted to your favorite flavors. Try chick peas instead of black beans and basil instead of cilantro.

TOTAL TIME: 15 MINUTES

Whisk together the lime juice, cilantro, and lime zest in a medium bowl. Whisk in the oil until well blended. Stir in the tuna, beans, pepper, and onion. Add the romaine lettuce and toss to coat. Serve immediately.

MAKES 2 SERVINGS

PER SERVING: 370 calories; 23 g total fat; 3 g saturated fat; 23 g carbohydrate; 5 g fiber; 23 g protein; 31 mg cholesterol; 395 mg sodium

---

METABOLISM BOOSTER: GO GREEN

Green tea is chock-full of antioxidants and has been linked to health benefits that range from protecting against cancer to improving your lipid profile.[1] Not only that, but drinking green tea has also been shown to boost metabolism. While it's true that the tea contains caffeine, its metabolism-revving properties aren't only due to this stimulant. This age-old beverage also contains compounds called catechins, which have been shown to stimulate thermogenesis—in simple terms, this means increasing your metabolism.[2] One study showed that people burned 180 more calories per day—with no increase in exercise or decrease in eating—just by adding three daily servings of green tea.[3] So start drinking up!

GREEK
TUNA SALAD

"THIS IS ONE of my favorite salads. The tuna and beans provide protein and fiber, and feta cheese is a daily food for me! I also love the strong taste of arugula . . . it adds to the flavor. If you are a fan of olives, add a few to this salad to pump up your MUFAs."

TOTAL TIME: 10 MINUTES

1. Combine the beans, tuna, artichoke hearts, cucumber, tomato, and oil in a medium bowl. Toss to blend well.
2. Divide the arugula among 4 plates. Divide the tuna mixture onto each and sprinkle each with 1 tablespoon of the cheese.

MAKES 4 SERVINGS

PER SERVING: 366 calories; 20 g total fat; 3 g saturated fat; 24 g carbohydrate; 5 g fiber; 28 g protein; 35 mg cholesterol; 410 mg sodium

1 can (15 ounces) no-sodium cannellini beans, rinsed and drained

1 can (14 ounces) low-sodium albacore tuna packed in water, drained

1 jar (14 ounces) marinated artichoke hearts, drained

½ cucumber, chopped

1 plum tomato, chopped

3 tablespoons olive oil

10 ounces arugula

¼ cup crumbled reduced-fat feta cheese

SLICED FENNEL AND BEET WITH SHRIMP

2 tablespoons orange juice concentrate

2 tablespoons white wine vinegar

¼ teaspoon salt

¼ teaspoon pepper

2 tablespoons extra virgin olive oil

12 ounces peeled and deveined, cooked large shrimp

4 cups mixed greens

1 bulb fennel

1 medium beet, peeled

2 ounces crumbled reduced-fat feta cheese

4 tablespoons chopped toasted walnuts

16 whole grain crispbreads

NO NEED TO clean the food processor between the fennel and beets. Just be sure to slice the fennel first so that the beet juice doesn't stain the fennel. Raw beets may be new to some folks, but give them a try. Crisp and sweet, these colorful veggies are delicious raw— try slicing or shredding in the food processor, which keeps your hands clean.

TOTAL TIME: 15 MINUTES

1. Whisk together the orange juice concentrate, vinegar, salt, and pepper in a medium bowl. Whisk in the oil. Remove 3 tablespoons of the vinaigrette to a small measuring cup. Add the shrimp to the bowl. Set both aside.

2. Divide the greens among 4 plates.

3. Thinly slice the fennel in a food processor (or very thinly slice). Divide among the plates, placing in a pile.

4. Change the cutting blade to the shredder. Shred the beet (cutting to fit if necessary) in the food processor. Divide among the plates, placing in another pile.

5. Arrange the shrimp on the plates. Drizzle with the dressing. Sprinkle each with one-quarter of the cheese and 1 tablespoon of the walnuts. Serve each with 4 crispbreads.

MAKES 4 SERVINGS

PER SERVING: 379 calories; 15 g total fat; 3 g saturated fat; 35 g carbohydrate; 5 g fiber; 26 g protein; 133 mg cholesterol; 529 mg sodium

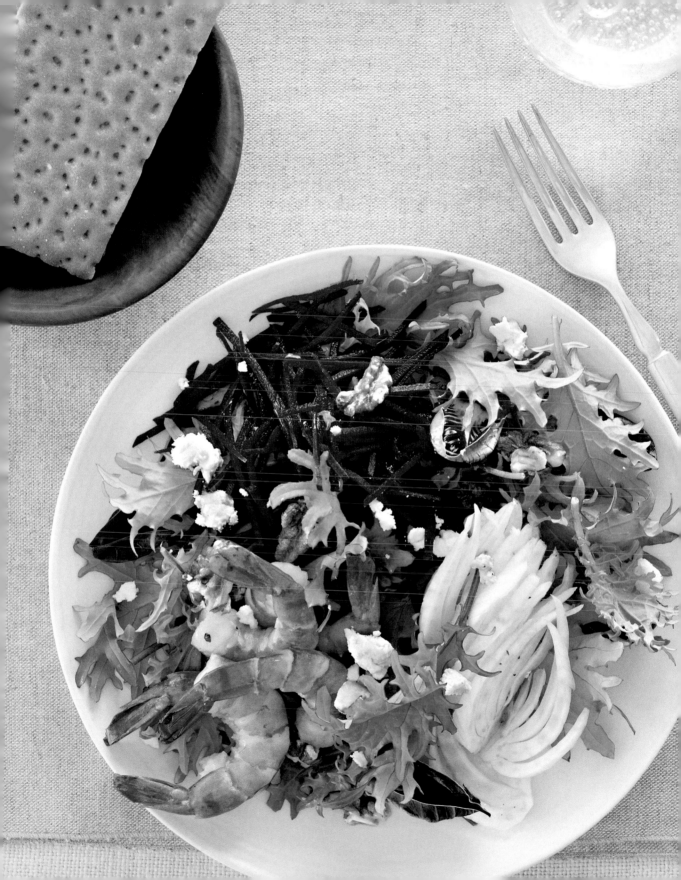

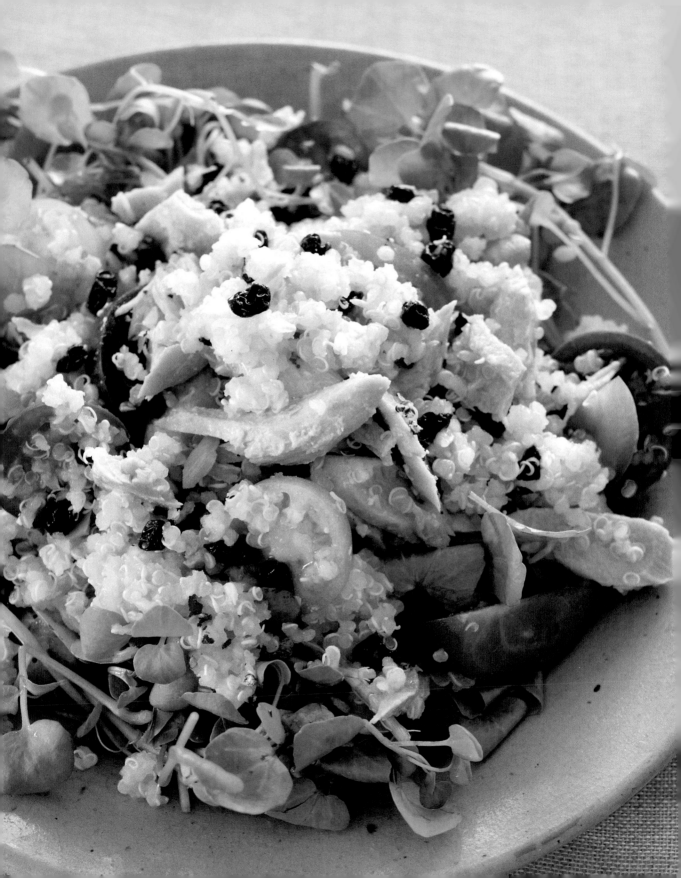

QUINOA
AND SALMON SALAD

QUINOA, PRONOUNCED "KEEN-WAH," produces its own natural insect repellent, called saponin. Great for warding off pests, saponin is quite bitter and gives quinoa a soapy taste. Rinse under cold running water until the water runs clear to remove all of the saponin and allow the mild, creamy flavor to come through.

TOTAL TIME: 25 MINUTES

1. Bring ⅔ cup water to a boil in a small saucepan. Add the quinoa and return to a boil. Reduce the heat to low, cover, and simmer for 15 minutes or until tender and the liquid has evaporated.

2. Meanwhile, whisk together the vinegar, honey, and pepper in a large bowl. Whisk in the oil until well blended. Stir in the tomatoes, currants or raisins, and warm quinoa.

3. Place the greens or watercress on 2 salad plates. Top with the quinoa mixture and salmon.

MAKES 2 SERVINGS

PER SERVING: 430 calories; 19 g total fat; 4 g saturated fat; 44 g carbohydrate; 5 g fiber; 24 g protein; 36 mg cholesterol; 535 mg sodium

¼ cup quinoa, rinsed well

2 tablespoons balsamic vinegar

1 tablespoon honey

¼ teaspoon pepper

2 tablespoons olive oil

1 cup cherry tomatoes, halved

¼ cup currants or raisins

3 cups mixed baby greens or watercress

1 pouch (7.1 ounces) pink salmon, flaked

CHAPTER 5 ∘ LUNCHES

MEDITERRANEAN PASTA SALAD WITH SHRIMP

8 ounces whole grain penne pasta

¼ cup fat-free plain Greek-style yogurt

2 tablespoons reduced-fat mayonnaise

2 tablespoons chopped fresh basil or 2 teaspoons dried

2 tablespoons lemon juice

1 teaspoon lemon zest

1 clove garlic, minced

12 ounces peeled and deveined, cooked shrimp, fresh or frozen and thawed

1 cup cherry tomatoes, halved

1 cucumber, halved, seeded, and sliced

4 cups romaine lettuce

TO GET THE most juice from lemons, bring them to room temperature and roll them on the counter under your palm to soften the fruit and release the juices. Halve and squeeze.

TOTAL TIME: 15 MINUTES

1. Prepare pasta according to package directions. Drain and rinse under cold running water. Drain well.

2. Meanwhile, whisk together the yogurt, mayonnaise, basil, lemon juice, lemon zest, and garlic in a large serving bowl. Add the pasta, shrimp, tomatoes, cucumber, and lettuce, tossing to coat.

MAKES 4 SERVINGS

PER SERVING: 341 calories; 4 g total fat; 1 g saturated fat; 51 g carbohydrate; 4 g fiber; 27 g protein; 129 mg cholesterol; 202 mg sodium

GINGER BROCCOLI SLAW WITH TOFU

A QUICK WAY TO peel fresh ginger is to scrape the sides with a teaspoon, removing just the skin. Peeling will remove the flesh just beneath the skin, which is the most flavorful part.

TOTAL TIME: 10 MINUTES

Whisk together the orange juice concentrate, vinegar, ginger, soy sauce, and oil. Add the broccoli slaw, pepper, and tofu. Toss to coat well.

MAKES 2 SERVINGS

PER SERVING: 312 calories; 13 g total fat; 2 g saturated fat; 29 g carbohydrate; 7 g fiber; 21 g protein; 0 mg cholesterol; 512 mg sodium

2 tablespoons frozen orange juice concentrate, thawed

2 tablespoons rice vinegar

1 tablespoon grated fresh ginger

2 teaspoons reduced-sodium soy sauce

1 tablespoon toasted sesame oil

1 package (12 ounces) broccoli slaw

1 red bell pepper, cut into 2" strips and halved

1 package (8 ounces) smoked tofu, cut into thin strips

CHAPTER 5 ○ LUNCHES

TURKEY GRINDER

1 medium onion, thinly sliced

2 tablespoons balsamic vinegar

2 teaspoons honey, divided

1 teaspoon Dijon mustard

2 whole grain rolls (3 ounces each), sliced in half

5 ounces natural low-sodium turkey breast

2 leaves romaine lettuce

1 whole roasted red pepper, patted dry and cut into thin strips

NOT ALL DELI turkey is the same. Ask to see the nutrition labels to find the products with the lowest fat and sodium contents. You can also do your research online before heading to the supermarket.

TOTAL TIME: 15 MINUTES

1. Heat a small saucepan coated with cooking spray over medium heat. Add the onion and cook, stirring, for 5 minutes or until browned. Add the vinegar and 1 teaspoon of the honey, cover, and cook for 3 to 5 minutes or until very tender.

2. Stir together the mustard and the remaining 1 teaspoon of honey in a small bowl. Spread onto the bottoms of the rolls.

3. Divide the turkey, lettuce, red pepper, and onion among the rolls.

MAKES 2 SERVINGS

PER SERVING: 320 calories; 4 g total fat; 1 g saturated fat; 50 g carbohydrate; 7 g fiber; 22 g protein; 25 mg cholesterol; 835 mg sodium

NOTE: This recipe is a little high in sodium (you want to aim for no more than 600 to 650 milligrams per meal), so be sure to work this recipe into your daily total of 2,300 milligrams of sodium by selecting recipes for the remaining meals that are around 300 to 400 milligrams each.

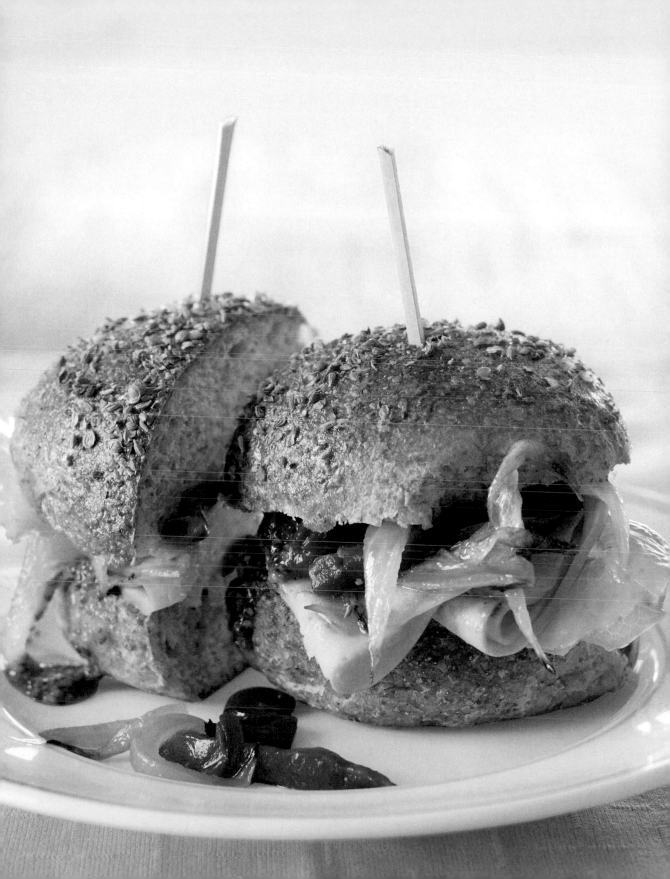

INDIAN SPICED TURKEY WRAP

¼ cup fat-free plain Greek-style yogurt

2 tablespoons chopped cilantro

½ teaspoon ground cumin

⅛ teaspoon salt

3 drops hot-pepper sauce

1 small zucchini, shredded

½ bell pepper, cut into thin strips and halved

2 whole grain tortillas (8" diameter, about 120 calories each)

2 tablespoons prepared mango chutney

6 ounces sliced turkey breast

ALTHOUGH DELI ROAST turkey breast works well in this recipe, leftover turkey breast is a better bet, as it is much lower in sodium. Roasted turkey breast slices much easier when chilled.

TOTAL TIME: 20 MINUTES

1. Stir together the yogurt, cilantro, cumin, salt, and pepper sauce in a small bowl. Stir in the zucchini and pepper. Chill until ready to use.

2. Place the tortillas on a work surface. Spread each with 1 tablespoon chutney. Top with the turkey and zucchini slaw. Roll to eat.

MAKES 2 SERVINGS

PER SERVING: 325 calories; 5 g total fat; 1 g saturated fat; 36 g carbohydrate; 6 g fiber; 33 g protein; 71 mg cholesterol; 595 mg sodium

QUICK SANDWICH WRAP

"THESE QUICK WRAPS are great on the go. The cream cheese gives it a rich taste, and I love the crunch the sunflower seeds add." Change up the recipe by trying different wraps, including spinach and tomato.

TOTAL TIME: 5 MINUTES

Place the tortilla on a plate. Spread with the cream cheese and layer with the spinach, turkey, carrots, and sunflower seeds. Roll.

MAKES 1 SERVING

PER SERVING: 385 calories; 11 g total fat; 2 g saturated fat; 28 g carbohydrate; 4 g fiber; 42 g protein; 103 mg cholesterol; 302 mg sodium

1 whole grain tortilla (8" diameter, about 120 calories)

1 tablespoon low-fat cream cheese

½ cup baby spinach

4 ounces sliced turkey breast

2 tablespoons shredded carrots

1 tablespoon sunflower seeds

DIET DILEMMA: EATING ON THE GO

Problem: You're running late and you're starving, so you pull into the nearest fast-food restaurant. Sure, you know you shouldn't be eating the hamburger, fries, and shake, but you had no other options, right?

Solution: Don't wait until you're famished to find food. Treat weight loss like a job, and plan ahead. If you know you're going to be on the road or at work late, pack diet-friendly meals and snacks to bring with you. If you're prepared with healthy options, it'll be a lot easier to avoid the drive-thru or vending machine.

CURRY CHICKEN SALAD SANDWICH

¼ cup fat-free plain Greek-style yogurt

¼ cup low-fat mayonnaise

2 teaspoons fresh lime juice

¼ teaspoon ground ginger

½ to 1 teaspoon green curry paste

12 ounces cooked chicken, chopped (about 3 cups)

4 scallions, sliced

2 ribs celery, chopped

1 cup shredded romaine lettuce

2 carrots, shredded

½ small cucumber, thinly sliced

4 whole wheat pitas (8" diameter), tops cut off

CURRY PASTE, THE base of Thai curry dishes, is a blend of herbs and spices. Green curry paste is milder than red, but either can be used in this dish. When first starting to use curry paste, use the smallest amount called for, then taste before adding more.

TOTAL TIME: 15 MINUTES

Stir together the yogurt, mayonnaise, lime juice, ginger, and curry paste. Stir in the chicken, scallions, and celery. Divide the chicken mixture, lettuce, carrots, and cucumber among the pitas.

MAKES 4 SERVINGS

PER SERVING: 351 calories; 7 g total fat; 1 g saturated fat; 45 g carbohydrate; 16 g fiber; 39 g protein; 72 mg cholesterol; 263 mg sodium

CHICKEN QUESADILLA

FOUND IN THE condiment section of your supermarket, liquid smoke adds a rich, smoky flavor to dishes, especially barbecue sauces. It's a dieter's dream, as it adds great flavor without any calories or sodium.

TOTAL TIME: 25 MINUTES

1. Preheat the oven to 400°F. Place the tortillas on a baking sheet. Set aside.

2. Combine the tomato sauce, tomato paste, vinegar, honey, Worcestershire sauce, onion, and liquid smoke (if using) in a small saucepan. Bring just to a boil over medium-high heat. Reduce the heat to low. Simmer for 15 minutes or until thickened.

3. Meanwhile, stir together the buttermilk and cheese with a fork in a large bowl, pressing to mash some of the cheese. Add the lettuce and toss to coat.

4. Stir the chicken and scallions into the barbecue sauce. Divide onto one side of each tortilla. Fold the other half of each tortilla over the chicken mixture. Bake for 5 minutes or until heated through. Place the quesadillas on 4 plates and cut each into 4 wedges. Serve with the salad.

MAKES 4 SERVINGS

PER SERVING: 401 calories; 8 g total fat; 2 g saturated fat; 45 g carbohydrate; 5 g fiber; 35 g protein; 77 mg cholesterol; 481 mg sodium

4 whole grain tortillas (8″ diameter, about 120 calories each)

1 can (8 ounces) no-salt-added tomato sauce

2 tablespoons tomato paste

2 tablespoons apple cider vinegar

2 tablespoons honey

1 tablespoon Worcestershire sauce

½ small onion, grated

¼ teaspoon liquid smoke (optional)

½ cup low-fat buttermilk

¼ cup crumbled low-fat blue cheese

6 cups chopped romaine lettuce

12 ounces cooked chicken breast, shredded (about 3 cups)

3 scallions, sliced

CHICKEN AND FENNEL PIZZA

3 tablespoons rice wine vinegar

2 teaspoons agave nectar or honey

4 carrots, cut lengthwise into quarters

2 whole grain tortillas (8" diameter, about 120 calories each)

1 small bulb fennel, trimmed and sliced

1 small red onion, cut into thin wedges

1 large chicken breast (about 6 ounces), cut into thin strips

¼ cup reduced-fat blue cheese

THE PICKLED CARROTS make a healthy, crunchy side for pizzas and sandwiches. Try adding cauliflower, celery, or bell peppers to the mixture for a variety of pickled vegetable options. The pickled vegetables may be refrigerated for up to 3 days.

TOTAL TIME: 25 MINUTES

1. Whisk together the vinegar and nectar or honey in a shallow dish. Add the carrots, tossing to coat. Cover and chill until serving.

2. Preheat the oven to 400°F. Place the tortillas on a baking sheet. Set aside.

3. Coat a medium skillet with cooking spray. Cook the fennel and onion for 5 minutes or until lightly browned. Add the chicken and cook for 5 minutes or until no longer pink. Remove from the heat.

4. Divide the mixture onto the tortillas. Sprinkle evenly with the cheese. Bake for 5 minutes or until the cheese melts. Cut into wedges. Serve with the carrots.

MAKES 2 SERVINGS

PER SERVING: 370 calories; 9 g total fat; 3 g saturated fat; 46 g carbohydrate; 12 g fiber; 30 g protein; 57 mg cholesterol; 602 mg sodium

ROAST BEEF
AND PORTOBELLO PANINI

A PANINI OR SANDWICH press works well for making these sandwiches, although an indoor grill (such as a George Foreman) also does the trick. Place the sandwiches coated with cooking spray on the press or grill and instead of using the heavy pan, close the lid and press slightly. There's no need to turn the sandwiches.

TOTAL TIME: 25 MINUTES

1. Place the mushrooms and onion slices in a shallow bowl with 3 tablespoons of the vinaigrette, turning to coat. Let stand for 10 minutes.

2. Lay 2 slices of the bread on the work surface. Spread each with ½ teaspoon vinaigrette. Top each with half the roast beef, 1 onion slice, and 1 mushroom. Top each with ¼ cup baby spinach, 1 slice cheese, and the remaining bread slices.

3. Spray the top slices with cooking spray and place sprayed-side down onto a grill pan or skillet. Coat the top slices of bread with cooking spray. Place a heavy pan over the top of the sandwiches. Cook, turning once, for 4 minutes or until browned and the cheese is melted.

MAKES 2 SERVINGS

PER SERVING: 335 calories; 11 g total fat; 3 g saturated fat; 33 g carbohydrate; 6 g fiber; 26 g protein; 38 mg cholesterol; 773 mg sodium

NOTE: This recipe is a little high in sodium (you want to aim for no more than 600 to 650 milligrams per meal), so be sure to work this recipe into your daily total of 2,300 milligrams of sodium by selecting recipes for the remaining meals that are around 300 to 400 milligrams each.

2 large portobello mushrooms

½ large red onion, cut into two ½" slices

3 tablespoons + 1 teaspoon low-fat Italian vinaigrette

4 slices whole wheat bread

4 ounces deli roast beef

½ cup baby spinach

2 thick slices low-fat provolone cheese (1 ounce total)

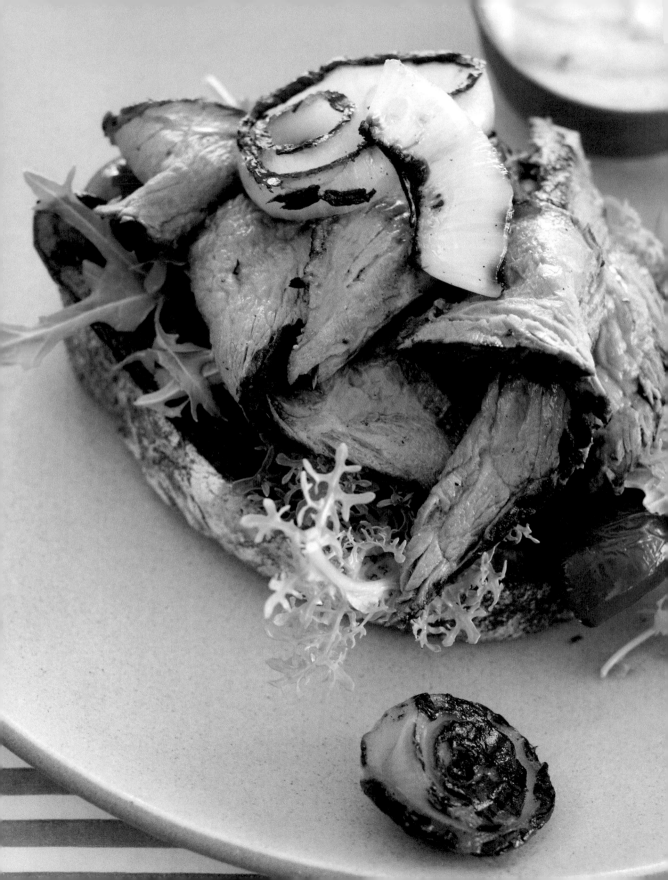

OPEN-FACE STEAK SANDWICH

FINDING A STEAK that's 12 ounces can be difficult, and if you do find one it will be quite thin, making cooking tricky. Your best bet is to buy a steak that's about 1½ pounds and cut it in half. Freeze one half in a freezer storage bag for up to 3 months.

TOTAL TIME: 30 MINUTES

1. Coat a grill rack or broiler pan with cooking spray. Preheat the grill or broiler. Press the black pepper onto the steak.

2. Whisk together the yogurt, oil, vinegar, horseradish, and honey until blended.

3. Grill or broil the steak, turning once, for 10 minutes or until a thermometer inserted into the center registers 145°F for medium-rare, 160°F for medium, or 165°F for well-done. Let stand for 10 minutes before slicing.

4. Coat the bell pepper and onion slices with cooking spray. Grill or broil, turning, for 8 minutes or until browned and tender. Slice the steak.

5. Place 1 bread slice on each of 4 plates. Top each with ½ cup mixed greens. Divide the onion, bell pepper, and steak among the 4 sandwiches. Drizzle with the horseradish vinaigrette.

MAKES 4 SERVINGS

PER SERVING: 376 calories; 13 g total fat; 4 g saturated fat; 39 g carbohydrate; 5 g fiber; 27 g protein; 40 mg cholesterol; 329 mg sodium

½ teaspoon freshly ground black pepper

12 ounces top round sirloin steak

¼ cup fat-free plain Greek-style yogurt

2 tablespoons olive oil

1 tablespoon white wine vinegar

1 tablespoon prepared horseradish

1 teaspoon honey

1 red bell pepper, quartered

1 large onion, cut into 4 thick slices

4 slices (1" thick, 2 ounces each) whole grain Italian bread

2 cups mixed greens

CHAPTER 5 ∘ LUNCHES

FISH PO' BOY
WITH CAJUN SLAW

3 tablespoons fat-free plain
  Greek-style yogurt

2 tablespoons reduced-fat
  mayonnaise

2 tablespoons agave
  nectar or honey

1 tablespoon cider vinegar

⅛ to ¼ teaspoon
  hot-pepper sauce

1 bag (14 ounces) pre-
  shredded coleslaw mix

1 red bell pepper, cut into
  1" strips, each halved

½ small onion, grated

2 teaspoons blackening
  seasoning

4 thick cod fillets
  (5 ounces each)

1 cup mixed greens

1 large tomato, thinly sliced

1 whole wheat baguette
  (12 ounces) slice
  lengthwise in half
  and cut crosswise
  into 4 pieces

THE PO' BOY is New Orleans's most famous sandwich—the submarine type, filled with fried meat or fish. Here, the flavorful fish is baked to keep the calories in check.

TOTAL TIME: 35 MINUTES

1. Preheat the oven to 350°F. Coat a baking sheet with cooking spray.

2. Whisk together the yogurt, mayonnaise, nectar or honey, vinegar, and hot-pepper sauce in a large bowl. Add the coleslaw mix, bell pepper, and onion. Toss to coat well. Chill until ready to serve.

3. Rub the seasoning over the fish. Place the fish on the baking sheet and bake, turning once, for 12 to 15 minutes or until the fish flakes easily.

4. Divide the greens and tomato on the baguettes. Top each with a fish fillet, folding fish to fit, if necessary. Serve with the coleslaw.

MAKES 4 SERVINGS

PER SERVING: 445 calories; 3 g total fat; 0 g saturated fat; 71 g carbohydrate; 8 g fiber; 36 g protein; 52 mg cholesterol; 775 mg sodium

NOTE: This recipe is a little high in sodium (you want to aim for no more than 600 to 650 milligrams per meal), so be sure to work this recipe into your daily total of 2,300 milligrams of sodium by selecting recipes for the remaining meals that are around 300 to 400 milligrams each.

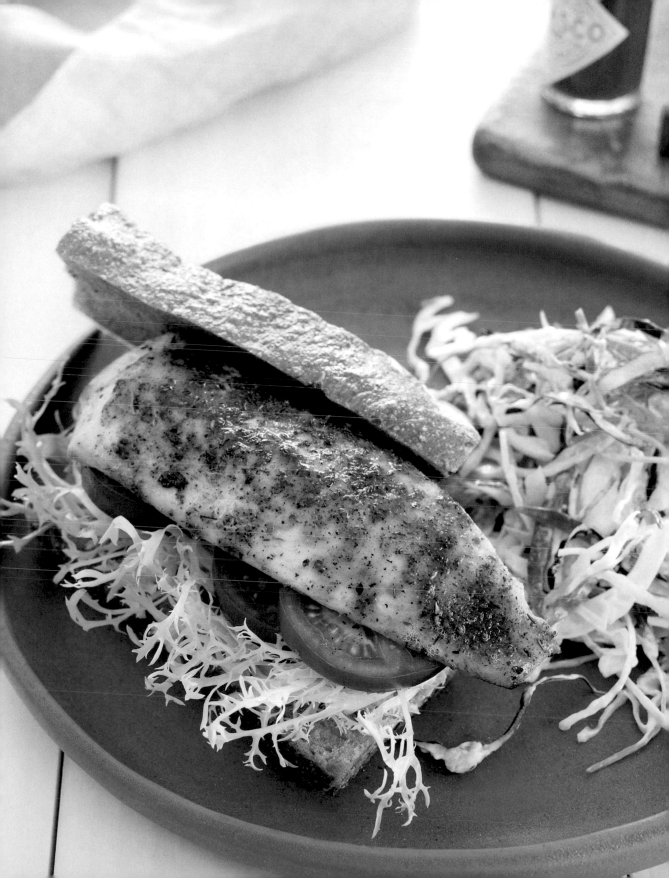

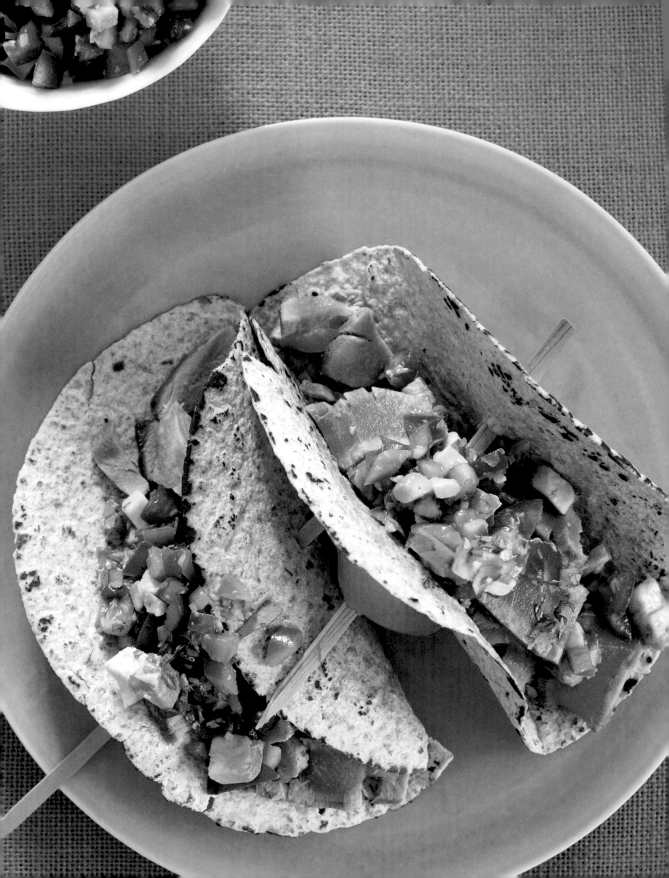

SEARED TUNA TACO WITH AVOCADO SALSA

S EARING IS COOKING meat or fish over high heat to create a brown coating. Avoid overcrowding the skillet, which reduces the temperature of the pan and creates steam—both will prevent proper searing.

TOTAL TIME: 20 MINUTES

1. Preheat the oven to 250°F. Combine the tomato, avocado, pepper, cilantro, 1 tablespoon lime juice, and salt in a small bowl. Set aside.

2. Wrap the tortillas in foil and place in the oven to warm.

3. Combine the cumin, garlic powder, and 1 teaspoon lime juice in a small bowl. Rub onto the tuna.

4. Heat a small skillet coated with cooking spray over high heat. Add the tuna and cook, turning once, for 3 to 6 minutes or until the fish is cooked to desired doneness. Slice.

5. Place each tortilla on a plate. Divide the tuna and tomato mixture on each. Fold and serve immediately.

MAKES 2 SERVINGS

PER SERVING: 403 calories; 21 g total fat; 3 g saturated fat; 26 g carbohydrate; 6 g fiber; 33 g protein; 43 mg cholesterol; 507 mg sodium

1 tomato, chopped

1 ripe avocado, halved, pitted, and chopped

½ green bell pepper, chopped

2 tablespoons chopped cilantro

1 tablespoon + 1 teaspoon lime juice

¼ teaspoon salt

2 whole grain tortillas (8" diameter, about 120 calories each)

1 teaspoon ground cumin

¼ teaspoon garlic powder

1 ahi tuna steak (8 ounces)

CHAPTER 5 ◦ LUNCHES

THAI SHRIMP WRAP

1 carrot, chopped

1 clove garlic

½" piece fresh ginger, peeled and coarsely chopped

2 tablespoons rice vinegar

2 tablespoons olive oil

2 large whole wheat tortillas (10" diameter)

1 cup shredded romaine lettuce

½ cup shredded red cabbage

½ small cucumber, thinly sliced

6 ounces peeled and deveined frozen shrimp, thawed

THIS SANDWICH COMES together in minutes using fully cooked frozen shrimp. If you have the foresight, place the shrimp in a sieve over a bowl and refrigerate the day before. This is the best way to thaw the shrimp, but if you're in a hurry, thaw in the microwave.

TOTAL TIME: 10 MINUTES

1. Combine the carrot, garlic, ginger, vinegar, and 2 tablespoons water in a food processor or blender. Puree until smooth. Gradually add the oil while the processor is running.

2. Lay the tortillas on a flat surface. Layer with the lettuce, cabbage, cucumber, and shrimp. Drizzle with the dressing. Roll.

MAKES 2 SERVINGS

PER SERVING: 309 calories; 15 g total fat; 2 g saturated fat; 27 g carbohydrate; 4 g fiber; 22 g protein; 166 mg cholesterol; 392 mg sodium

CARAMELIZED ONION AND SHRIMP PIZZA

CARAMELIZED ONION ADDS a rich decadence to this pizza. You can prepare the onion ahead of time and chill for up to 3 days. Reheat before stirring in the arugula.

TOTAL TIME: 20 MINUTES

1. Heat the oil in a small saucepan coated with cooking spray over medium heat. Add the onion and cook, stirring, for 5 minutes or until browned. Add the vinegar, cover, and cook for 10 minutes or until very tender. Remove from the heat.

2. Preheat the broiler. Place the pitas on a baking sheet.

3. Stir the arugula or spinach into the onion mixture and divide among the pitas. Top each with the shrimp and cheese.

4. Broil at least 5 inches from the heat source for 3 minutes or until the cheese melts.

MAKES 4 SERVINGS

PER SERVING: 327 calories; 13 g total fat; 3 g saturated fat; 22 g carbohydrate; 7 g fiber; 36 g protein; 182 mg cholesterol; 380 mg sodium

2 tablespoons olive oil

1 large onion, thinly sliced

2 tablespoons balsamic vinegar

4 whole wheat pitas (8" diameter)

2 cups baby arugula or spinach

12 ounces peeled and deveined cooked shrimp

4 ounces light Jarlsberg cheese, shredded

ZESTY TOFU "EGG" SALAD

1 package (12 ounces drained weight) extra-firm low-fat tofu

3 tablespoons mayonnaise

2 tablespoons fat-free plain Greek-style yogurt

2 tablespoons prepared mango chutney

2 teaspoons curry powder

¼ teaspoon salt

2 scallions, chopped

1 carrot, shredded

1 rib celery, finely chopped

¼ cup raisins

8 slices whole wheat bread, toasted

1 large tomato, sliced

2 cups mixed greens

FOR A FASTER way to release the liquid from firm tofu, place it in a clean, non-terry dish towel. Wrap the towel around the tofu, twisting the ends while holding it over a bowl or the sink. Firmly wring out the liquid. Continue with step 2 of this recipe.

TOTAL TIME: 20 MINUTES

1. Remove the tofu from the package and drain. Place in a colander in the sink. Place a flat plate on top of the tofu and a heavy can of vegetables on the plate for 15 minutes to drain.

2. Meanwhile, whisk together the mayonnaise, yogurt, chutney, curry powder, and salt. Stir in the scallions, carrot, celery, and raisins. Crumble the tofu and add to the bowl. Toss gently to coat.

3. Place 1 slice of bread on each of 4 plates. Top each with some tomato slices, ½ cup greens, and one-quarter of the tofu mixture. Top with the remaining bread slices.

MAKES 4 SERVINGS

PER SERVING: 274 calories; 4 g total fat; 1 g saturated fat; 45 g carbohydrate; 6 g fiber; 15 g protein; 0 mg cholesterol; 682 mg sodium

NOTE: This recipe is a little high in sodium (you want to aim for no more than 600 to 650 milligrams per meal), so be sure to work this recipe into your daily total of 2,300 milligrams of sodium by selecting recipes for the remaining meals that are around 300 to 400 milligrams each.

GRILLED VEGETABLE WRAP

HAILING FROM PROVENCE, traditional aioli is a creamy sauce of oil and garlic thickened with egg. Here we've used yogurt in place of the egg and added basil for a fresh, delicious flavor.

TOTAL TIME: 25 MINUTES

1. To make the aioli, whisk together the yogurt, basil, oil, vinegar, and salt until well blended. Chill.

2. To make the wraps, coat the grill rack or broiler pan with cooking spray. Preheat the grill or broiler.

3. Coat the onion, pepper, and zucchini with cooking spray. Grill or broil the vegetables 4" from the heat, turning once, for 10 minutes or until tender.

4. Place 1 wrap on each of 4 plates. Top each with ½ cup arugula, one-quarter of the vegetables, and one-quarter of the tofu. Drizzle with 2 tablespoons of the basil aioli. Roll and serve.

MAKES 4 SERVINGS

PER SERVING: 373 calories; 15 g total fat; 2 g saturated fat; 41 g carbohydrate; 9 g fiber; 22 g protein; 0 mg cholesterol; 653 mg sodium

NOTE: This recipe is a little high in sodium (you want to aim for no more than 600 to 650 milligrams per meal), so be sure to work this recipe into your daily total of 2,300 milligrams of sodium by selecting recipes for the remaining meals that are around 300 to 400 milligrams each.

BASIL AIOLI

½ cup fat-free plain Greek-style yogurt

2 tablespoons minced fresh basil

1 tablespoon extra virgin olive oil

1 tablespoon balsamic vinegar

¼ teaspoon salt

WRAPS

1 large red onion, cut into 4 slices

1 red bell pepper, cut into 4 thick slices

1 small zucchini, cut lengthwise into 4 slices

4 whole grain wraps or tortillas (8" diameter, about 120 calories each)

2 cups baby arugula or mixed greens

12 ounces smoked baked tofu

lickety-split lunches

15 quick and easy lunches

Whether you work at home or go to an office, making time to prepare a sensible lunch will keep you on track and feeling satisfied until snack time. Many traditional lunches, like a 6-inch pastrami sandwich, take-out burger and fries, or even a take-out salad bathed in heavy dressing, will use up most of your daily calorie allotment. Using some simple tips, the following recipes turn classic lunch favorites into delicious waist-whittling meals in under 15 minutes.

The 2-Week Turnaround lunch should contain 400 calories broken down as 1 grain/starchy veggie, 1 protein, 2 veggies, and 1 fat. Below are some techniques used throughout this chapter to keep calories down and boost flavor. Each can be used in your own creations as well.

SWITCH OUT THE MAYO. Fat-free Greek-style plain yogurt and low-fat sour cream are rich, creamy bases that when combined with flavorful items such as pesto or chutney make a delicious sandwich spread without all the fat in mayonnaise. You can even add some vinegar to create a low-fat salad dressing. Occasionally, you'll want a smear of mayo, and when you do, reach for the low-fat mayo, which will save you quite a bit of calories.

GO FOR WHOLE GRAIN. There are so many whole wheat and whole grain choices available these days that it makes selecting the best ones a bit confusing. Using the ingredient and nutrition labels will ensure you select the best option every time. First, be sure the word *whole* is listed—look for whole wheat flour and not just wheat flour. Next, look at the grams of fiber. A good source of fiber contains 2.5 to 4.9 grams of fiber.[4] Some breads, rolls, tortillas, and pitas will contain as many as 6 to 8 grams, and as you know by now, the more the better. Finally, look at the calories, as they vary considerably, and go for the lowest. For example, there are 8-inch tortillas as low as 80 calories while others are 200 calories.

SEASON IT WITH SALAD DRESSING. The supermarket shelves of bottled salad dressings can certainly be overwhelming. But if you take some time to locate the reduced-fat ones that offer unique but bold flavor, you'll be able to throw together some chopped veggies and leftover chicken or fish and have a great meal in minutes. Just be sure to select ones with minimal sodium.

TURKEY BURGER

4 ounces (99% fat-free) ground turkey breast

1 cup shredded lettuce

1 roasted red pepper, patted dry and sliced

½ avocado, cut into slices

2 tablespoons reduced-fat lime vinaigrette

½ whole wheat pita (8" diameter)

1. Shape the turkey into a burger and grill or broil for 8 minutes or until a thermometer inserted into the center registers 165°F and the meat is no longer pink.

2. Arrange the lettuce on a plate. Top with the burger, pepper, and avocado slices. Drizzle with the vinaigrette. Serve with the pita.

MAKES 1 SERVING

PER SERVING: 405 calories; 18 g total fat; 2 g saturated fat; 33 g carbohydrate; 7 g fiber; 34 g protein; 45 mg cholesterol; 534 mg sodium

CHUTNEY TURKEY SALAD

4 tablespoons prepared mango chutney, chopped

⅓ cup light sour cream

1 tablespoon white wine vinegar

1 chunk (12 ounces) deli turkey breast, chopped

1 red bell pepper, chopped

1 mango, peeled, pitted, and chopped

4 cups baby or chopped romaine lettuce

4 small whole grain rolls

1. Stir together the chutney, sour cream, and vinegar in a large bowl. Add the turkey, pepper, and mango. Toss to coat well.

2. Line 4 plates with the lettuce and divide the turkey salad among the plates. Serve with the rolls.

MAKES 4 SERVINGS

PER SERVING: 369 calories; 5 g total fat; 2 g saturated fat; 49 g carbohydrate; 7 g fiber; 33 g protein; 77 mg cholesterol; 338 mg sodium

nutrition notes

● WHILE AVOCADOS *seem almost too rich and delicious to be good for you, they're actually one of the best natural sources of monounsaturated fat, the good kind of fat that is associated with heart health.*

● MANGOES *are rich in beta-carotene, which enhances the immune system and plays a role in cancer prevention (particularly lung, esophagus, and stomach cancer).*

nutrition notes

● PHYTOCHEMICALS ("phyto" means plant) are the biologically active compounds in plants that define their color and flavor. Red tomatoes get their hue from the phytochemical lycopene, and studies suggest that lycopene-rich diets reduce the risk of certain cancers, including prostate cancer.

● CANNED FRUITS, like mandarin oranges, are harvested and canned at their peak, and although the high-heat canning process destroys some of the vitamins, most of the nutrients remain. Just be sure to use canned fruit with no added sugar.

ITALIAN BLT SANDWICH

2 teaspoons reduced-fat mayonnaise

2 teaspoons refrigerated reduced-fat pesto

1 sandwich flatbread (about 100 calories), split

¼ cup arugula or 2 large lettuce leaves

½ small vine-ripened tomato, sliced

3 slices cooked turkey bacon, halved crosswise

1 carrot, cut into sticks

Spread the mayonnaise and pesto on one side of the bread. Top with the arugula or lettuce, tomato, bacon, and other side of the bread. Cut in half and serve with the carrot sticks.

MAKES 1 SERVING

PER SERVING: 309 calories; 14 g total fat; 1 g saturated fat; 27 g carbohydrate; 12 g fiber; 30 g protein; 81 mg cholesterol; 558 mg sodium

ASIAN CHICKEN SALAD

2 cups mixed salad greens

3 ounces cooked chicken breast, shredded (about ¾ cup)

½ cup cooked brown rice

¼ cup mandarin oranges

2 tablespoons low-fat sesame-ginger salad dressing

2 tablespoons sliced toasted almonds

Combine the greens, chicken, rice, oranges, and dressing in a medium bowl. Sprinkle with the almonds.

MAKES 1 SERVING

PER SERVING: 393 calories; 12 g total fat; 2 g saturated fat; 40 g carbohydrate; 6 g fiber; 34 g protein; 72 mg cholesterol; 487 mg sodium

CHICKEN WALDORF SALAD

2 teaspoons olive oil

2 teaspoons red wine vinegar

¼ teaspoon pepper

3 ounces cooked chicken breast
   (about ¾ cup)

1 cup spinach

2 ribs celery, chopped

1 small apple, chopped

¼ cup whole wheat croutons

1 tablespoon chopped walnuts

Whisk together the oil, vinegar, and pepper in a medium bowl. Stir in the chicken, spinach, celery, apple, croutons, and walnuts.

MAKES 1 SERVING

PER SERVING: 436 calories; 18 g total fat; 3 g saturated fat; 38 g carbohydrate; 9 g fiber; 32 g protein; 72 mg cholesterol; 685 mg sodium

NOTE: This recipe is a little high in sodium (you want to aim for no more than 600 to 650 milligrams per meal), so be sure to work this recipe into your daily total of 2,300 milligrams of sodium by selecting recipes for the remaining meals that are around 300 to 400 milligrams each.

nutrition notes

● GREENS, *such as spinach, blow boring iceberg away. They're loaded with vitamins A, C, and K, as well as folate, potassium, magnesium, iron, lutein, and phytochemicals.*

DIET DILEMMA: EMOTIONAL EATING

Problem: When you're sad, do you reach for the ice cream or chips? You're not alone. Many people (especially women) do this—it's called emotional eating. Emotional eating is when you eat for comfort, not for hunger. How can you tell if you have emotional hunger versus actual, physical hunger? Emotional hunger normally comes on suddenly, while physical hunger is more gradual. And emotional hunger feels like it needs to be satisfied instantly, but physical hunger can wait.

Solution: Try to address your feelings head-on, rather than treating them with food. If you can, figure out what you're sad or angry about—maybe you can't fix it, but sometimes just acknowledging the problem can help. Look beyond food for comfort—call a friend, take a walk, or watch a funny movie.

SWEET POTATO SALAD

1¾ pounds sweet potatoes, peeled and cut into ¾" cubes

1 pound cooked chicken breast, chopped (about 3¾ cups)

½ jar (12 ounces) roasted red peppers, drained, patted dry, and cut into ½" pieces

2 cups chopped arugula or baby arugula

¼ cup low-fat creamy Italian salad dressing

1. Place the potatoes in a large microwaveable bowl. Cover and microwave on high for 8 minutes or until tender; cool to room temperature.

2. Add the chicken, peppers, arugula, and dressing. Toss to coat well.

MAKES 4 SERVINGS

PER SERVING: 354 calories; 5 g total fat; 1 g saturated fat; 37 g carbohydrate; 7 g fiber; 38 g protein; 96 mg cholesterol; 416 mg sodium

SALMON SALAD

¼ cup whole grain couscous

1 tablespoon olive oil

1 tablespoon balsamic vinegar

1 tablespoon Dijon mustard

⅛ teaspoon black pepper

3 ounces cooked salmon fillets

½ small cucumber, sliced

1 carrot, shredded

1. Prepare the couscous according to package directions.

2. Whisk together the oil, vinegar, mustard, pepper, and 1 teaspoon water in a medium bowl. Add the couscous, salmon, cucumber, and carrot, tossing to coat well.

MAKES 1 SERVING

PER SERVING: 417 calories; 20 g total fat; 3 g saturated fat; 37 g carbohydrate; 7 g fiber; 24 g protein; 47 mg cholesterol; 433 mg sodium

STEAK FAJITA

1 whole grain tortilla
(8″ to 10″ diameter)

1 small onion, cut into wedges

1 cup frozen mixed peppers, thawed

3 ounces cooked, sliced
top round steak

½ cup prepared salsa

1 tablespoon reduced-fat sour cream

1. Place the tortilla on a plate. Set aside.

2. Heat a small skillet coated with cooking spray over medium heat. Cook the onion for 5 minutes or until browned. Add the peppers and cook for 3 minutes or until heated through. Place on the tortilla.

3. Heat the steak in the same skillet for 2 minutes or just until heated. Place on top of the pepper mixture.

4. Top with the salsa and sour cream.

MAKES 1 SERVING

PER SERVING: 392 calories; 10 g total fat; 3 g saturated fat; 38 g carbohydrate; 3 g fiber; 33 g protein; 71 mg cholesterol; 679 mg sodium

NOTE: This recipe is a little high in sodium (you want to aim for no more than 600 to 650 milligrams per meal), so be sure to work this recipe into your daily total of 2,300 milligrams of sodium by selecting recipes for the remaining meals that are around 300 to 400 milligrams each.

SHRIMP AND GRAPEFRUIT SALAD

2 cups mixed greens

3 ounces peeled and deveined,
cooked large shrimp

½ cup jarred grapefruit segments

½ cup grape tomatoes

3 tablespoons low-fat bottled lime
or balsamic vinaigrette

1 ounce whole wheat crackers

Place the greens on a plate. Top with the shrimp, grapefruit, and tomatoes. Drizzle with the dressing and serve with the crackers.

MAKES 1 SERVING

PER SERVING: 370 calories; 14 g total fat; 2 g saturated fat; 42 g carbohydrate; 6 g fiber; 23 g protein; 166 mg cholesterol; 689 mg sodium

NOTE: This recipe is a little high in sodium (you want to aim for no more than 600 to 650 milligrams per meal), so be sure to work this recipe into your daily total of 2,300 milligrams of sodium by selecting recipes for the remaining meals that are around 300 to 400 milligrams each.

nutrition notes

● BEEF *is packed with lots of good-for-you, high-quality protein and nutrients, but if you don't choose the right cut, it can also provide a hefty dose of artery-clogging saturated fat. Round steaks and roasts (including top round, eye round, bottom round, and round tip), as well as tenderloin, sirloin, and chuck shoulder, are all good picks.*

● GRAPEFRUITS *are very high in vitamin C, which helps support the immune system and promotes cardiovascular health.*

CHAPTER 5 ◦ LUNCHES

nutrition notes

● ALTHOUGH RED BELL PEPPERS *and hot peppers are members of the same family, bell peppers have a lot less capsaicin, the compound that gives peppers their heat. Red peppers are packed with vitamin C (they have even more than oranges) and the potent antioxidant vitamin E.*

● A STAPLE *in the Middle East, bulgur is a whole grain that is extremely high in fiber.*

CRAB SALAD SANDWICH

1 can (6 ounces) crabmeat, drained

2 tablespoons low-fat mayonnaise

2 teaspoons lemon juice

½ to 1 teaspoon prepared horseradish

1 rib celery, chopped

4 large lettuce leaves

1 whole wheat pita, cut in half and split open

1 red bell pepper, cut into sticks

Toss together the crabmeat, mayonnaise, lemon juice, horseradish, and celery in a medium bowl. Place the lettuce in the pita halves. Divide the crabmeat mixture between the pitas. Serve with the pepper sticks.

MAKES 2 SERVINGS

PER SERVING: 232 calories; 7 g total fat; 1 g saturated fat; 21 g carbohydrate; 4 g fiber; 22 g protein; 81 mg cholesterol; 594 mg sodium

WHITE BEAN AND BULGUR SALAD

2 tablespoons bulgur

1 tablespoon olive oil

2 tablespoons balsamic vinegar

⅛ teaspoon salt

3 ounces smoked tofu, cut into strips

¼ cup reduced-sodium white beans, rinsed and drained

1 tomato, chopped

1 green bell pepper, chopped

¼ cup chopped basil

1. Prepare the bulgur according to package directions.

2. Whisk together the oil, vinegar, salt, and black pepper to taste in a large bowl. Add the bulgur, tofu, beans, tomato, bell pepper, and basil. Toss to coat well.

MAKES 1 SERVING

PER SERVING: 418 calories; 19 g total fat; 3 g saturated fat; 43 g carbohydrate; 11 g fiber; 20 g protein; 0 mg cholesterol; 609 mg sodium

TUNA MELT

1 tablespoon olive oil

1½ tablespoons balsamic vinegar

Pinch of black pepper

1 cup shredded lettuce

½ cup chopped red bell pepper

2 tablespoons fat-free plain
Greek-style yogurt

3 ounces canned tuna packed
in water, drained

2 scallions, chopped

1 slice whole grain bread

1 slice provolone cheese

1. Preheat the broiler.

2. Whisk together the oil, vinegar, and black pepper in a medium bowl. Remove 1 tablespoon to a large bowl.

3. Add the lettuce and bell pepper to the large bowl. Toss to coat.

4. Stir the yogurt into the medium bowl with the remaining vinegar mixture. Stir in the tuna and scallions. Spread onto the bread and top with the cheese. Broil for 3 minutes or until browned. Serve with the lettuce mixture.

MAKES 1 SERVING

PER SERVING: 420 calories; 21 g total fat; 5 g saturated fat; 24 g carbohydrate; 5 g fiber; 32 g protein; 55 mg cholesterol; 583 mg sodium

nutrition notes

● LIKE CANNED SALMON, *canned tuna is a great, inexpensive source of healthy omega-3 fats. For the highest omega-3 levels, choose albacore tuna packed in water.*

TOFU TOMATO SALAD

1½ cups mixed greens

3 ounces smoked tofu, cut into ½" cubes

½ cup grape or cherry tomatoes, halved

1 scallion, sliced

2 tablespoons chopped cilantro

2 teaspoons olive oil

2 teaspoons lime juice

4 rye crispbreads

1. Place the greens on a plate.

2. Combine the tofu, tomatoes, scallion, cilantro, oil, and lime juice in a small bowl. Toss to coat well. Place over the greens. Serve with the crispbreads.

MAKES 1 SERVING

PER SERVING: 351 calories; 14 g total fat; 2 g saturated fat; 41 g carbohydrate; 10 g fiber; 17 g protein; 0 mg cholesterol; 328 mg sodium

VEGETARIAN STUFFED POTATO

1 medium leftover baked potato

3 tablespoons fat-free milk

½ cup steamed broccoli, chopped

1 carrot, shredded

3 ounces smoked tofu, chopped

2 tablespoons shredded sharp Cheddar cheese

1. Preheat the oven to 350°F. Slice the potato lengthwise in half. Scoop out the pulp and place in a small bowl. Place the skins on a baking sheet.

2. Heat a small skillet coated with cooking spray over medium heat. Add the pulp and milk, mashing with a fork to blend. Cook for 2 minutes. Stir in the broccoli and carrot and cook for 2 minutes or until heated. Remove from the heat and stir in the tofu.

3. Spoon the potato mixture into the skins. Sprinkle with the cheese and bake for 5 minutes or until heated through.

MAKES 1 SERVING

PER SERVING: 394 calories; 10 g total fat; 4 g saturated fat; 55 g carbohydrate; 9 g fiber; 23 g protein; 13 mg cholesterol; 400 mg sodium

VEGGIE BURGER

1 frozen veggie burger

1½ tablespoons reduced-fat mayonnaise

½ whole wheat English muffin

1 cup shredded romaine lettuce

1 tomato, chopped

1 small peach, sliced

1 tablespoon balsamic vinegar

2 teaspoons olive oil

1. Prepare the veggie burger according to package directions. Spread the mayonnaise on the muffin and top with the burger.

2. Meanwhile, toss together the lettuce, tomato, peach, vinegar, oil, and salt and pepper to taste in a medium bowl. Serve with the burger.

MAKES 1 SERVING

PER SERVING: 405 calories; 17 g total fat; 2 g saturated fat; 49 g carbohydrate; 13 g fiber; 18 g protein; 0 mg cholesterol; 695 mg sodium

NOTE: This recipe is a little high in sodium (you want to aim for no more than 600 to 650 milligrams per meal), so be sure to work this recipe into your daily total of 2,300 milligrams of sodium by selecting recipes for the remaining meals that are around 300 to 400 milligrams each.

nutrition notes

● BY CHOOSING A VEGGIE BURGER *instead of a traditional ground beef hamburger, you're saving tons of calories and fat grams—while still getting the "feel" of eating a burger.*

DINNERS

CHAPTER 6 ∘ DINNERS

"ALL MEN SEEK
ONE GOAL:
SUCCESS OR
HAPPINESS."

—ARISTOTLE

TURKEY LONDON BROIL WITH CHIMICHURRI

1 boneless, skinless turkey breast (1½ pounds)

1 tablespoon olive oil, divided

½ teaspoon ancho chili powder

½ teaspoon mild smoked paprika

1 cup brown rice

1 can (15 ounces) black beans

¾ cup parsley

¾ cup cilantro

3 tablespoons fresh lime juice

1 tablespoon sliced pickled jalapeño

¾ teaspoon dried oregano

½ teaspoon salt

3 cloves garlic, rinsed and drained

DON'T BE ALARMED by the name—turkey London broil is simply a boneless, skinless turkey breast that's been split to cook quickly and evenly. Cook this lean protein in the oven (see below) or grill indirectly over medium heat for 1 hour, turning every 15 minutes.

TOTAL TIME: 1 HOUR 10 MINUTES

1. Preheat the oven to 350°F.

2. Place the turkey breast in a roasting pan. Drizzle the turkey with 1 teaspoon of the oil and rub to coat. Sprinkle on the chili powder and paprika, and rub over turkey until evenly coated.

3. Bake the turkey for 50 to 60 minutes, or until a thermometer inserted into the thickest portion registers 165°F and the juices run clear. Let stand for 5 minutes.

4. Meanwhile, prepare the rice according to package directions.

5. Remove from the heat and stir in the beans. While the rice cooks, process the garlic in a blender or food processor until finely chopped. Add the parsley and cilantro; process until finely chopped. Add the lime juice, jalapeño, oregano, salt, the remaining 2 teaspoons olive oil, and ½ cup water. Process until blended.

6. Serve the turkey drizzled with the sauce along with the rice and beans.

MAKES 6 SERVINGS

PER SERVING: 338 calories; 7 g total fat; 1 g saturated fat; 34 g carbohydrate; 5 g fiber; 34 g protein; 70 mg cholesterol; 459 mg sodium

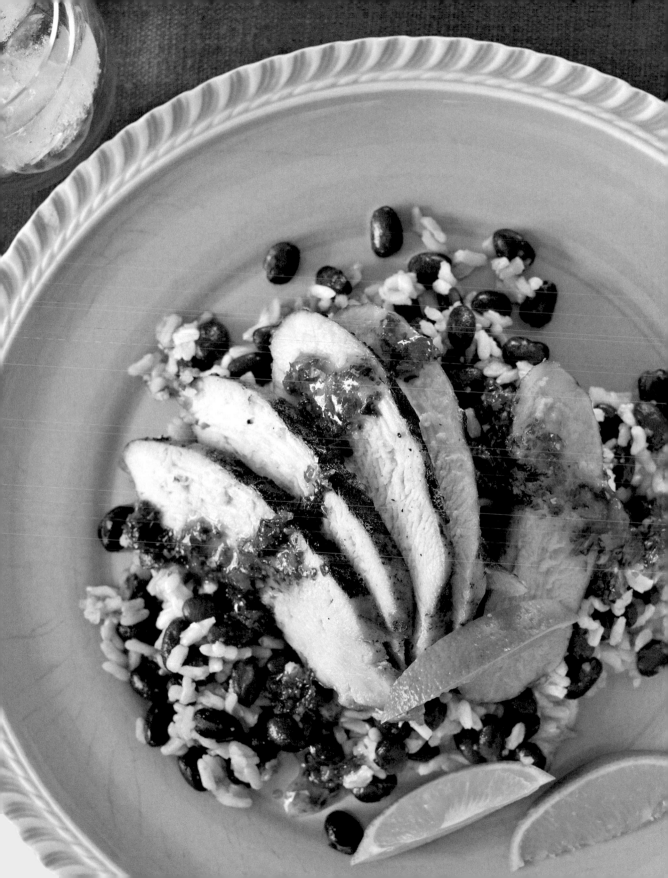

TURKEY CUTLETS WITH MASHED SWEET POTATOES

1¾ pounds sweet potatoes, peeled and cut into ¾" cubes

3 tablespoons orange marmalade spreadable fruit

¼ cup + 2 tablespoons reduced-fat cream cheese, divided

¼ teaspoon salt

1½ teaspoons olive oil

4 turkey cutlets (1 pound)

2 large shallots, halved and thinly sliced

½ cup reduced-sodium chicken broth

2 tablespoons maple syrup

1 tablespoon balsamic vinegar

1 tablespoon spicy brown mustard

2 tablespoons chopped parsley (optional)

1 package (12 ounces) micro-steam sugar snap peas

SEASON THIS SAUCE with your favorite flavored mustard, such as coarse grain, horseradish, or honey mustard. Pork or chicken cutlets would be a great substitute for the turkey.

TOTAL TIME: 30 MINUTES

1. Place the sweet potatoes in a large microwaveable bowl. Microwave, covered, on high for 8 minutes or until tender. (Do not drain.) Add the spreadable fruit, ¼ cup of the cream cheese, and salt. Mash until well blended.

2. Meanwhile, heat the oil in a nonstick skillet over medium heat. Cook the turkey, turning once, for 6 to 8 minutes or until browned and the juices run clear. Transfer the cutlets to a plate.

3. Add the shallots to the skillet and cook, stirring, for 2 minutes or until softened and golden. Stir in the broth, syrup, vinegar, and mustard. Bring to a simmer and cook for 2 minutes. Stir in the remaining 2 tablespoons cream cheese until blended. Add the turkey and cook for 1 minute or until heated through. Sprinkle with the parsley.

4. Microwave the peas according to the package directions.

5. Divide the turkey, sweet potatoes, and sugar snap peas among 4 plates.

MAKES 4 SERVINGS

PER SERVING: 423 calories; 7 g total fat; 3 g saturated fat; 54 g carbohydrate; 7 g fiber; 36 g protein; 58 mg cholesterol; 491 mg sodium

TURKEY FENNEL SAUTÉ

L EEKS ARE GROWN in sand, which ends up between each layer. The quickest way to remove the sand is to slice each leek in half lengthwise and run each half under cold water while separating the layers and rinsing off all of the sand.

TOTAL TIME: 35 MINUTES

1. Prepare the couscous according to package directions. Place in a bowl and stir in 1 tablespoon of the oil. Set aside.

2. Meanwhile, heat the remaining 2 tablespoons of the oil in a large nonstick skillet over medium heat. Cook the leeks, fennel, pepper, and garlic for 10 minutes, stirring, until lightly browned. Sprinkle with the salt.

3. Stir in the turkey and cook for 3 minutes or until the turkey is no longer pink. Stir in the broth, spinach, and lemon juice and cook for 1 minute or until the spinach wilts.

4. Divide the couscous among 4 plates. Divide the turkey mixture over the couscous.

MAKES 4 SERVINGS

PER SERVING: 407 calories; 13 g total fat; 1 g saturated fat; 44 g carbohydrate; 9 g fiber; 36 g protein; 45 mg cholesterol; 325 mg sodium

1 cup whole wheat couscous

3 tablespoons olive oil, divided

2 leeks, sliced

2 bulbs fennel, sliced

1 red bell pepper, sliced

2 cloves garlic, minced

¼ teaspoon salt

1 pound turkey tenderloin, sliced into ½" strips

¼ cup low-sodium chicken broth

4 cups baby spinach

1 tablespoon fresh lemon juice

CHAPTER 6 ○ DINNERS

CHICKEN WITH QUINOA PILAF

3 tablespoons olive oil, divided

1 cup quinoa

1 onion, chopped

2 cloves garlic, minced

2 cups low-sodium chicken broth

4 cups Swiss chard or spinach, tough stems removed and chopped

2 tablespoons chopped fresh basil

½ teaspoon salt, divided

4 boneless, skinless chicken breast halves (4 ounces each)

¼ teaspoon pepper

A GOOD SOURCE OF vitamins A and C, Swiss Chard, also called Chard, is a cruciferous vegetable related to beets. Choose bunches with bright green leaves and crisp stalks.

TOTAL TIME: 45 MINUTES

1. Coat a medium saucepan with cooking spray. Heat 2 tablespoons of the oil over medium-high heat. Add the quinoa, onion, and garlic, and cook for 5 minutes or until lightly browned. Add the broth, chard, basil, and ¼ teaspoon of the salt. Bring to a boil. Reduce the heat to low, cover, and simmer, stirring twice, for 15 minutes or until the quinoa is tender and the liquid is absorbed.

2. Meanwhile, sprinkle the chicken with the pepper and the remaining ¼ teaspoon salt. Heat the remaining 1 tablespoon oil in a large nonstick skillet over medium heat. Cook the chicken, turning once, for 8 minutes or until a thermometer inserted in the thickest portion registers 160°F and the juices run clear.

3. Divide the chicken and quinoa pilaf among 4 plates.

MAKES 4 SERVINGS

PER SERVING: 411 calories; 15 g total fat; 2 g saturated fat; 33 g carbohydrate; 4 g fiber; 36 g protein; 66 mg cholesterol; 481 mg sodium

SAUSAGE LASAGNA

"A TIP I GOT from an Italian friend long ago—that there's no need to ever precook lasagna noodles—changed my opinion of lasagna. I hated cooking the noodles first. The turkey sausage and cheese make this a hearty, satisfying dish. Great in cool weather and perfect for a large group!"

TOTAL TIME: 1 HOUR 40 MINUTES

1. Preheat the oven to 375°F. Coat a 13″ × 9″ baking dish with cooking spray.

2. Heat the oil in a medium saucepan over medium heat. Cook the sausage and garlic, stirring often, for 8 minutes or until browned. Add the pasta sauce and bring to a simmer. Reduce the heat to low and simmer for 5 minutes.

3. Meanwhile, in a medium bowl, stir together the ricotta, basil, egg, pepper, 1 cup of the mozzarella cheese, and ¾ cup Parmesan.

4. Spread 1½ cups of the sauce on the bottom of the baking dish. Arrange 3 noodles over the sauce. Layer with one-third of the ricotta mixture, one-third of the spinach, one-third of the remaining sauce, 1 cup mozzarella, and ⅓ cup Parmesan. Repeat the layers 2 more times, ending with the cheese on top.

5. Coat a piece of foil with cooking spray and cover the dish. Bake for 40 minutes. Remove the foil and bake uncovered for 20 minutes, or until a knife inserted in the center comes out hot. Let stand for 15 minutes before serving.

6. Cut into 12 rectangles and serve each with ½ cup of the romaine.

MAKES 12 SERVINGS

PER SERVING: 379 calories; 16 g total fat; 9 g saturated fat; 27 g carbohydrate; 2 g fiber; 31 g protein; 69 mg cholesterol; 727 mg sodium

NOTE: This recipe is a little high in sodium (you want to aim for no more than 600 to 650 milligrams per meal), so be sure to work this recipe into your daily total of 2,300 milligrams of sodium by selecting recipes for your remaining meals that have around 300 to 400 milligrams each.

1 tablespoon olive oil

1 pound low-fat turkey sausage

2 cloves garlic, minced

2 jars (24 to 26 ounces total) fat-free, low-sodium pasta sauce

1 container (15 ounces) part-skim ricotta cheese

¼ cup chopped basil

1 egg

¼ teaspoon pepper

4 cups shredded part-skim mozzarella cheese, divided

1¾ cup grated Parmesan cheese, divided

9 whole grain lasagna noodles

1 bag (6 ounces) spinach, chopped

6 cups romaine lettuce

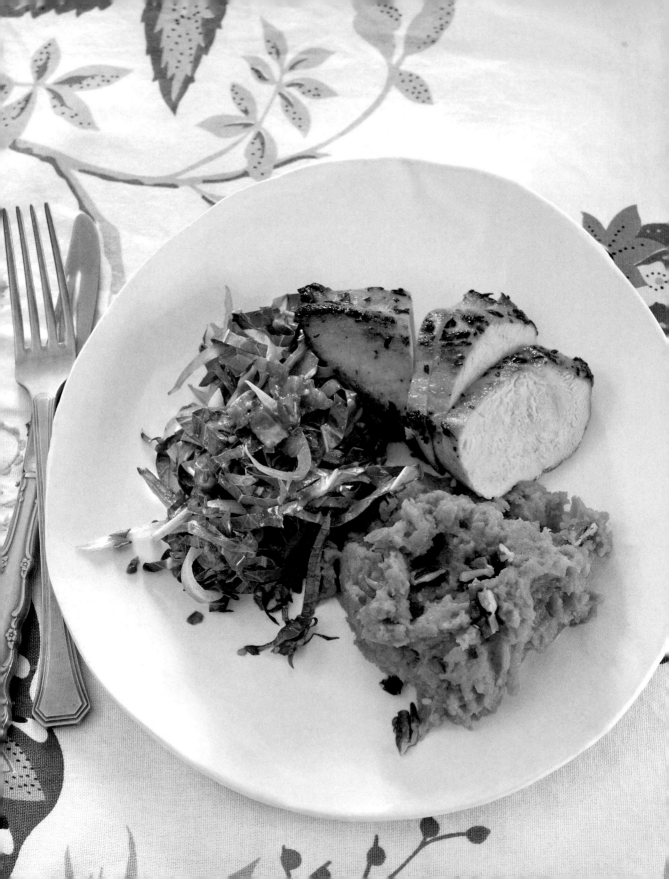

CHICKEN WITH SWEET POTATOES AND COLLARD GREENS

SWEET POTATOES ARE chockful of beta-carotene; opt for the darkest ones, as they have the most vitamins. Often you'll see sweet potatoes labeled "yams" in grocery stores. True yams are not even related to sweet potatoes, and are available mostly in Latin markets. Yams don't have the same sweet flavor as sweet potatoes.

TOTAL TIME: 45 MINUTES

1. Preheat the oven to 375°F. Coat a large baking sheet with cooking spray; set aside. Coat a baking dish with cooking spray.

2. Place the sweet potatoes cut-side down in the baking dish. Bake for 30 minutes, or until tender. Peel the sweet potatoes and place them in a medium bowl. Mash with the olive oil, black pepper and ¼ teaspoon of the salt. Stir in the pecans.

3. Place the chicken breasts in the baking dish and rub with the garlic, rosemary, and ¼ teaspoon of the salt. Bake for 15 to 20 minutes, or until a thermometer inserted in the thickest portion registers 160°F and the juices run clear.

4. Meanwhile, place the collard greens, tomatoes, onion, and oregano on the baking sheet and coat them with cooking spray. Toss and spread out on the sheet. Bake with the chicken for 15 minutes. Sprinkle with the vinegar and the remaining ¼ teaspoon salt. Return to the oven and bake for 5 minutes.

5. Divide the chicken, sweet potatoes, and collard greens among 4 plates.

MAKES 4 SERVINGS

PER SERVING: 340 calories; 14 g total fat; 2 g saturated fat; 24 g carbohydrate; 6 g fiber; 30 g protein; 66 mg cholesterol; 561 mg sodium

2 medium (5 ounces each) sweet potatoes, cut in half

2 tablespoons olive oil

¼ teaspoon black pepper

¾ teaspoon salt, divided

¼ cup pecans, chopped

4 boneless, skinless chicken breast halves (4 ounces each)

2 cloves garlic, finely minced

1 tablespoon finely chopped rosemary

4 cups sliced collard greens

4 tomatoes, chopped

1 onion, thinly sliced

1 tablespoon chopped fresh oregano

2 tablespoons cider vinegar

CHAPTER 6 ◦ DINNERS

BRAISED CHICKEN WITH TOMATO, EGGPLANT, AND OLIVES

6 ounces whole wheat penne pasta

2 tablespoons olive oil, divided

4 large plum tomatoes, chopped

4 cups thinly sliced Japanese eggplant

1 onion, thinly sliced

3 cloves garlic, minced

¼ cup chopped, fresh mixed herbs, such as basil or thyme

½ teaspoon salt

1 pound boneless, skinless chicken breasts, cut into 1" strips

¼ cup pitted kalamata olives

¼ cup low-sodium chicken broth

JAPANESE AND ASIAN eggplants have a mild flavor and tender flesh. Look for the thin, straight varieties with purple, striated, or light-colored skin. Baby eggplant may be substituted.

TOTAL TIME: 30 MINUTES

1. Prepare the pasta according to package directions. Remove from the heat and stir in 1 tablespoon of the oil.

2. Meanwhile, heat the remaining 1 tablespoon oil in a large skillet over medium-high heat. Add the tomatoes, eggplant, onion, garlic, herbs, and salt. Cook, stirring, for 10 minutes, or until the vegetables are tender.

3. Add the chicken, olives, and broth and cook for 5 minutes, or until the chicken is no longer pink and the juices run clear.

4. Divide the pasta among 4 plates. Top with the chicken mixture.

MAKES 4 SERVINGS

PER SERVING: 408 calories; 11 g total fat; 2 g saturated fat; 43 g carbohydrate; 8 g fiber; 345 g protein; 66 mg cholesterol; 562 mg sodium

GRILLED CHICKEN AND POBLANO TACOS

POBLANO PEPPERS ADD a nice, mild heat to these tacos. If you like, use a green bell pepper in place of the poblanos and serve with hot sauce. Place the prepared taco ingredients on a large platter for a self-serve meal. This recipe is easily halved to serve 2.

TOTAL TIME: 40 MINUTES

1. Slice the scallions, keeping the white and green parts separate. Place the white parts in a resealable bag. Add the salsa, chili powder, and chicken breasts and seal, pushing out the air. Knead the bag to evenly coat the chicken. Marinate, refrigerated, for 30 minutes.

2. In a large bowl, whisk the mayonnaise, vinegar, honey, cumin, and salt, Add the cabbage, ¼ cup of the cilantro, and half of the scallion greens; toss to coat well.

3. Preheat the grill or heat a grill pan over medium-high heat. Grill the peppers, turning occasionally, for 6 minutes, or until tender-crisp. Grill the chicken, turning once, for 12 minutes, or until a thermometer inserted in the thickest portion registers 160°F and the juices run clear. Let stand for 5 minutes.

4. Meanwhile, wrap the tortillas in paper towels. Microwave on high for 1 minute or until warmed. Slice the chicken into strips.

5. Place 2 corn tortillas on each of 4 plates. Divide the chicken, peppers, avocado, and remaining cilantro and scallion greens among the tortillas. Serve with the cabbage slaw.

MAKES 4 SERVINGS

PER SERVING: 382 calories; 9 g total fat; 2 g saturated fat; 45 g carbohydrate; 8 g fiber; 32 g protein; 66 mg cholesterol; 554 mg sodium

4 scallions

¼ cup prepared salsa

2 teaspoons chili powder

1 pound boneless, skinless chicken breasts

¼ cup + 2 tablespoons reduced-fat mayonnaise

2 tablespoons rice wine vinegar

2 tablespoons honey

½ teaspoon ground cumin

½ teaspoon salt

6 cups thinly sliced napa cabbage (about 1 pound)

½ cup chopped cilantro, divided

2 poblano peppers, seeded and cut in half

8 corn tortillas

½ ripe avocado, diced

CHAPTER 6 ○ DINNERS

CHICKEN AND GREEN BEAN SHEPHERD'S PIE

1 pound Yukon gold potatoes, scrubbed and cut into 2" cubes

4 tablespoons olive oil, divided

¾ teaspoon salt, divided

1 large onion, finely chopped

12 ounces chicken tenders, cut into ¼" strips

8 ounces green beans, cut into 1" pieces

12 ounces white mushrooms, sliced

3 cups torn spinach

¼ cup reduced-fat sour cream

¼ teaspoon black pepper

IF YOU DON'T have an ovenproof skillet or for a special presentation, you may transfer the hot mixture to a 10" baking dish. Continue cooking as instructed. To make ahead, assemble the dish and refrigerate for up to 2 days. Increase the baking time to 45 minutes.

TOTAL TIME: 1 HOUR

1. Preheat the oven to 375°F.

2. Place the potatoes in a steamer basket set in a pan of boiling water over medium heat. Cover and cook for 15 minutes, or until very tender. Place in a medium bowl with 2 tablespoons of the oil and ¼ teaspoon of the salt. Mash until smooth.

3. Meanwhile, heat the remaining 2 tablespoons oil in a large ovenproof skillet over medium-high heat. Cook the onion and chicken, stirring, for 5 minutes, or until the chicken is no longer pink and the juices run clear.

4. Stir in the green beans, mushrooms, spinach, sour cream, pepper, and the remaining ½ teaspoon salt.

5. Cover with the mashed potatoes. Bake for 35 minutes, or until hot in the center. Turn the oven to broil and broil 4" to 6" from the heat for 3 to 5 minutes, or until the tops of the potatoes are browned.

MAKES 4 SERVINGS

PER SERVING: 360 calories; 15 g total fat; 2 g saturated fat; 31 g carbohydrate; 6 g fiber; 27 g protein; 51 mg cholesterol; 545 mg sodium

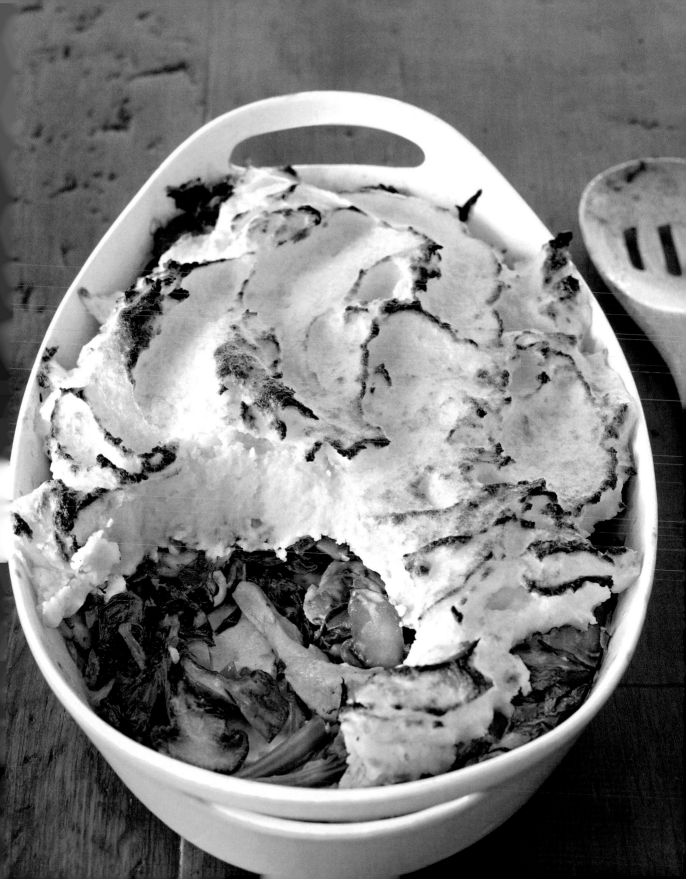

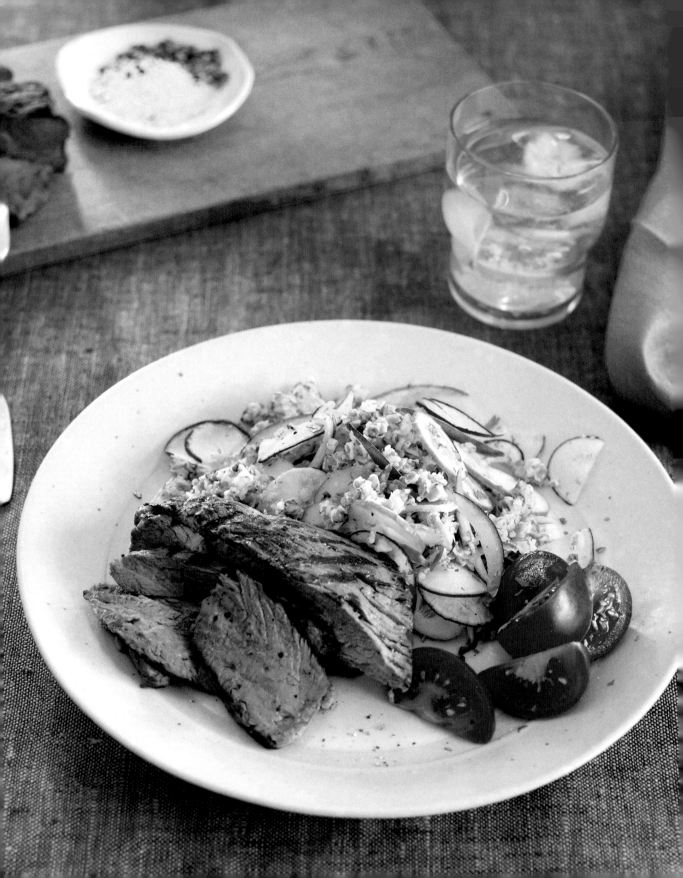

STEAK
WITH BULGUR SALAD

ECHNICALLY A FRUIT, tomatoes are usually referred to as a vegetable. Whatever you call them, they are a delicious addition to any healthy meal. Never refrigerate tomatoes of any kind. The cold will destroy their flavor.

TOTAL TIME: 45 MINUTES

1. Place the bulgur in a medium bowl. Cover with 1 cup boiling of water. Fluff with a fork and let sit for 10 minutes, or until the water is absorbed.

2. Meanwhile, in a large bowl, combine the tomatoes, onion, vinegar, oil, radishes, cucumber, parsley, pepper, and ½ teaspoon of the salt. Once the bulgur is ready, gently stir it into the tomato mixture.

3. Coat a skillet with cooking spray and heat over medium heat. Sprinkle the steak with the remaining ¼ teaspoon salt and cook in the skillet, turning once, for 6 to 8 minutes, or until a thermometer inserted in the center registers 145°F for medium-rare, 160°F for medium, or 165°F for well-done.

4. Remove the steak to a cutting board and let stand for 10 minutes. Slice the steak and place it on a large platter with the salad.

MAKES 4 SERVINGS

PER SERVING: 402 calories; 13 g total fat; 3 g saturated fat; 40 g carbohydrate; 9 g fiber; 31 g protein; 53 mg cholesterol; 530 mg sodium

1 cup bulgur (cracked wheat)

4 tomatoes, each cut into 8 wedges

2 tablespoons chopped red onion

¼ cup red wine vinegar

2 tablespoons olive oil

5 radishes, sliced

1 cucumber, sliced

1 cup fresh parsley, chopped

¼ teaspoon pepper

¾ teaspoon salt, divided

16-ounce sirloin steak, trimmed of all visible fat

CHAPTER 6 · DINNERS

TERIYAKI FLANK STEAK WITH SHIITAKE SAUTÉ

6 teapoons rice or white wine vinegar

2 garlic cloves, chopped

⅓ cup + 2 teaspoons reduced-sodium teriyaki sauce, divided

2 tablespoons finely chopped fresh ginger, divided

1 tablespoon + 2 teaspoons canola oil, divided

1 flank steak (1 pound) trimmed

¾ pound shiitake mushrooms, stems discarded and caps whole (halved, if large)

2 large shallots, thinly sliced

1 package (16 ounces) frozen sugar snap peas

1 teaspoon toasted sesame oil

½ small whole wheat baguette (4 ounces), diagonally sliced

IF YOU LIKE, serve this with 2 cups of a cooked wild rice mixture instead of the baguette. Leftovers can be made into a salad, served atop mixed greens, dotted with cherry tomatoes, and drizzled with reduced-fat Asian sesame dressing.

TOTAL TIME: 25 MINUTES PLUS STANDING TIME

1. Combine vinegar, garlic, ⅓ of the teriyaki sauce, 5 teaspoons of the ginger, and 1 tablespoon canola oil in a resealable bag. Add the steak, push out all the air, and seal. Refrigerate for 1 to 24 hours.

2. Preheat a grill or broiler to medium-high heat. Grill or broil the steak, turning once, for 12 to 15 minutes, or until a thermometer inserted in the center registers 145°F for medium-rare, 160°F for medium, or 165°F for well-done. Let stand for 10 minutes before slicing.

3. Meanwhile, heat the remaining 2 teaspoons canola oil in a large nonstick skillet over medium-high heat. Add the mushrooms and shallots and cook for 5 minutes, stirring frequently. Add the peas and cook for 3 minutes, stirring occasionally. Stir in the remaining 1 teaspoon of ginger and cook for 30 seconds. Remove from the heat and stir in the sesame oil and the remaining 2 teaspoons teriyaki sauce.

4. Thinly slice the flank steak. Serve with the mushroom mixture and baguette.

MAKES 4 SERVINGS

PER SERVING: 387 calories; 14 g total fat; 3 g saturated fat; 32 g carbohydrate; 6 g fiber; 34 g protein; 37 mg cholesterol; 686 mg sodium

NOTE: This recipe is a little high in sodium (you want to aim for no more than 600 to 650 milligrams per meal), so be sure to work this recipe into your daily total of 2,300 milligrams of sodium by selecting recipes for your remaining meals that have around 300 to 400 milligrams each.

STUFFED FLANK STEAK

"THIS IS DEFINITELY a regular family favorite! Full of flavor and once again, when the spinach cooks down, its mild flavor is okay with my kids." Switch out the asparagus for any seasonal vegetable your family enjoys.

TOTAL TIME: 1 HOUR

1. Preheat the broiler. Line a baking sheet with aluminum foil and coat with cooking spray. Cut six 12" pieces of kitchen twine.

2. Lay the flank steak on a cutting board with the grain of the steak running vertically in front of you. With a sharp knife held parallel to the board, cut the steak in half, stopping 1" from the edge of the steak. (You can also ask your butcher to butterfly the steak for you.) Open the cut steak like a book and turn it sideways, so the grain is running horizontally.

3. Layer the spinach, cheese, and garlic on the steak, leaving a 1" border all around. Roll up the steak from the long edge, shaping it into a log. Starting 1½" from one end, tie the meat with the twine at 1½" intervals. Place it on the baking sheet.

4. Rub with the oil and sprinkle with the salt and pepper. Broil 4" from the heat, turning once, for 10 to 15 minutes, or until browned and a thermometer inserted in the center registers 145°F for medium-rare, 160°F for medium, or 165°F for well-done. Let stand for 10 minutes before slicing.

5. Cut the steak into 12 slices. Place 2 slices on each of 6 plates with a potato topped with 2 tablespoons of the yogurt and ⅙ of the asparagus.

MAKES 6 SERVINGS

PER SERVING: 334 calories; 11 g total fat; 4 g saturated fat; 34 g carbohydrate; 5 g fiber; 27 g protein; 38 mg cholesterol; 406 mg sodium

---

1 flank steak (1 pound), trimmed

1 bag (7 ounces) baby spinach

½ cup Parmesan cheese

2 cloves garlic, minced

1 tablespoon olive oil

½ teaspoon salt

¼ teaspoon pepper

6 medium russet potatoes, baked

¾ cup fat-free plain Greek-style yogurt

1½ pounds asparagus, trimmed and steamed

CHAPTER 6 ○ DINNERS

BRAISED BEEF WITH GREENS AND BULGUR

1 pound beef sirloin, cut into 1½" cubes

2 tablespoons olive oil

1 onion, chopped

2 cups reduced-sodium beef broth, divided

2 red bell peppers, chopped

2 tablespoons fresh oregano

1 bay leaf

½ teaspoon salt, divided

4 cups mustard greens, tough stems removed and leaves chopped

1 cup bulgur (cracked wheat)

½ cup chopped Italian parsley

MUSTARTD GREENS HAVE a peppery flavor and are a favorite in southern cooking. The dark green leaves are an excellent source of vitamins A and C, thiamine, and riboflavin. Delicious steamed, sautèed, roasted, or added to soups and stews, include mustard greens in your meals.

TOTAL TIME: 1 HOUR 20 MINUTES

1. Heat a Dutch oven or large stockpot over medium-high heat. Cook the beef, working in batches if necessary. Turn the cubes for 5 minutes or until browned on all sides. Remove to a bowl and set aside.

2. Add the oil to the pot and heat over medium-high heat. Cook the onions for 5 minutes, stirring.

3. Add 1 cup of the broth, stirring to break up any browned bits. Add the beef, peppers, oregano, bay leaf, and ¼ teaspoon of the salt. Bring to a simmer. Reduce the heat to low, cover, and simmer for 15 minutes. Add the mustard greens and cook for 15 minutes, or until the beef is tender.

4. Meanwhile, place the bulgur and the remaining ¼ teaspoon salt in a medium bowl. Cover with the remaining 1 cup broth. Fluff with a fork and let stand for 10 minutes or until the water is absorbed. Stir in the parsley.

5. Divide the beef mixture among 4 bowls. Top each with ¼ of the bulgur.

MAKES 4 SERVINGS

PER SERVING: 391 calories; 12 g total fat; 3 g saturated fat; 38 g carbohydrate; 11 g fiber; 34 g protein; 50 mg cholesterol; 615 mg sodium

MEATLOAF BURGER WITH HOMEMADE KETCHUP

THIS BURGER IS served open-face. You may think that making your own ketchup is silly, but this one is so much more delicious and unique from purchased ketchup, it's well worth the effort. Store it in the refrigerator for up to 1 week.

TOTAL TIME: 35 MINUTES

1. Place the tomatoes, molasses, agave nectar, cinnamon, 2 tablespoons of the vinegar, and ¼ teaspoon of the salt in a medium saucepan over medium heat. Bring the mixture to a simmer and cook for 15 minutes. Place in a blender or food processor and puree until smooth. Return to the pan and cook for 20 minutes, or until reduced by half. Chill until ready to serve.

2. Meanwhile, in a large bowl, combine the cabbage, oil, pepper, the remaining 2 tablespoons cider vinegar, and ⅛ teaspoon of the salt. Toss to coat well. Chill until ready to serve.

3. In a large bowl, combine the onion, bread crumbs, egg, mustard, beef, and the remaining ⅛ teaspoon salt until well blended. Shape the mixture into 4 patties.

4. Heat a large nonstick skillet coated with cooking spray over medium heat. Cook the red onion slices for 8 minutes, or until browned, turning once. Remove to a plate.

5. Recoat the skillet with cooking spray and cook the burgers, turning once, for 8 minutes, or until a thermometer inserted in the center registers 160°F and the meat is no longer pink.

6. Place half of a bun on each of 4 plates. Top with a burger, onion slice, and the ketchup. Serve with the cabbage on the side.

MAKES 4 SERVINGS

PER SERVING: 435 calories; 15 g total fat; 4 g saturated fat; 42 g carbohydrate; 7 g fiber; 33 g protein; 123 mg cholesterol; 529 mg sodium

---

2 tomatoes, chopped

1 tablespoon molasses

2 teaspoons agave nectar or honey

¼ teaspoon cinnamon

4 tablespoons cider vinegar, divided

½ teaspoon salt, divided

4 cups shredded cabbage

2 tablespoons olive oil

¼ teaspoon black pepper

1 onion, minced

1 cup whole wheat panko bread crumbs

1 egg

⅛ teaspoon dry ground mustard

1 pound 95% lean ground beef

4 thick slices red onion

2 whole wheat hamburger buns, split in half

CHAPTER 6 • DINNERS

BEEF AND VEGETABLE STEW WITH GARLICKY GRITS

STEW

1 tablespoon olive oil

12 ounces top round beef, cut into 1" cubes

8 shallots, minced

1 onion, cut into wedges

2 cloves garlic, minced

½ cup red wine or beef broth

2 cups baby carrots

1 potato, cut into 1" chunks

1½ teaspoons dried basil

1½ teaspoons dried oregano

3 cups low-sodium beef broth

½ teaspoon salt

GRITS

5 cloves garlic, minced

⅓ cup quick corn grits

2 tablespoons olive oil

¼ teaspoon salt

A FAVORITE IN SOUTHERN cooking, grits are typically stone-ground hominy— although technically, any ground grain, including corn, oats, or rice— is considered grits. As a general rule, when boiling grits, use 5 parts water or fat-free milk to 1 part grits.

TOTAL TIME: 1 HOUR 15 MINUTES

TO MAKE THE STEW

1. Heat the oil in a Dutch oven or large saucepan over medium-high heat. Cook the beef, turning often, for 5 minutes, or until browned. Remove to a bowl.

2. Reduce the heat to medium and add the shallots, onion, and garlic to the same pot. Cook, stirring occasionally, for 5 minutes, or until browned.

3. Add the wine or broth and cook for 2 minutes, stirring to release the browned bits. Add the beef, carrots, potato, basil, oregano, broth, salt, and 2 cups of water. Bring to a boil. Reduce the heat to medium and simmer for 45 minutes, or until the potato and carrots are tender.

TO MAKE THE GRITS

1. Heat a nonstick saucepan coated with cooking spray over medium heat. Cook the garlic, stirring constantly, for 2 minutes, or until lightly browned. Add 2 cups of water to the saucepan and bring to a boil. Whisk in the grits, olive oil, and salt. Reduce the heat to low, and cook, whisking frequently, for 5 minutes, or until the water is absorbed and the grits are tender.

2. Divide the grits among 4 large bowls or soup plates. Top with the stew.

MAKES 4 SERVINGS

PER SERVING: 426 calories; 16 g total fat; 3 g saturated fat; 39 g carbohydrate; 3 g fiber; 28 g protein; 55 mg cholesterol; 284 mg sodium

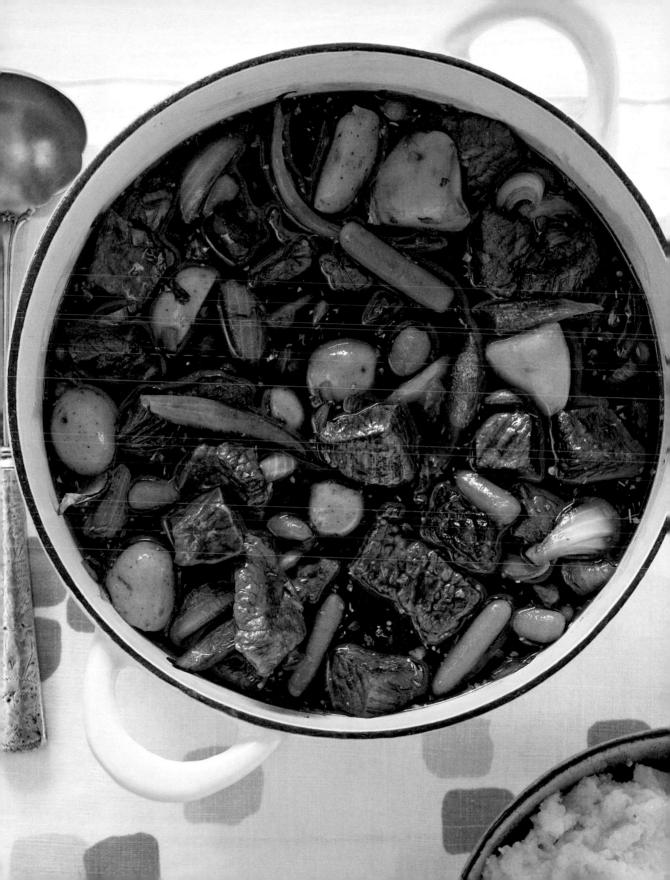

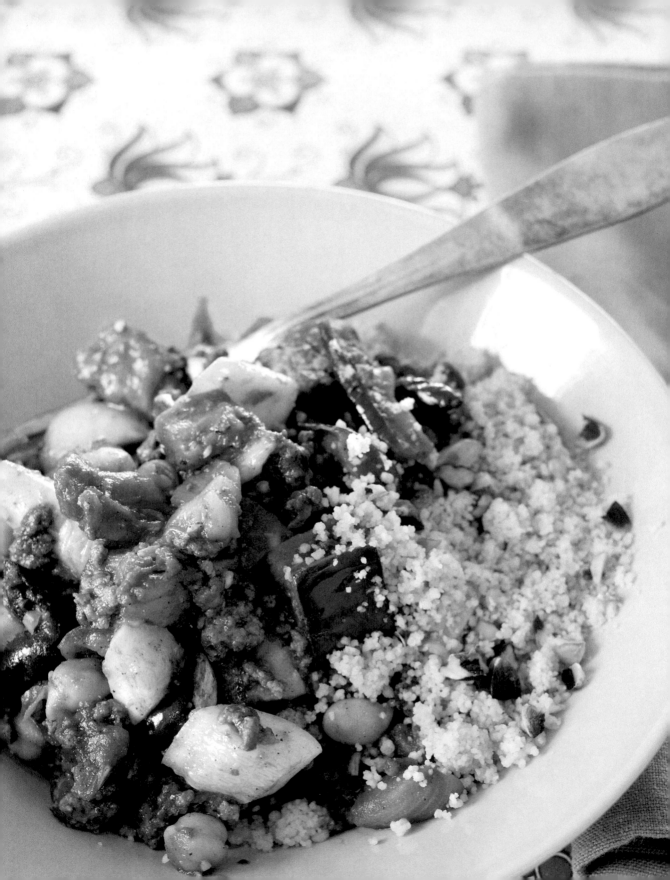

BEEF AND EGGPLANT TAGINE

THIS TASTY MOROCCAN dish would be just as delicious made with ground chicken or turkey breast or crumbled soy sausage in place of the beef. For a one-dish meal, omit the couscous and increase the chickpeas to 2 cups.

TOTAL TIME: 45 MINUTES

1. Heat a large nonstick saucepan or deep skillet coated with cooking spray over medium-high heat. Add the beef and cook for 6 to 8 minutes, or until no longer pink, stirring and breaking up the meat with the side of a spoon. Transfer to a bowl and set aside.

2. Heat the oil in the same skillet. Add the eggplant and cook for 5 minutes, stirring occasionally. Add the squash, garlic, garam masala, cinnamon, and ginger. Cook, stirring frequently, for 1 minute, or until the spices are fragrant and toasted.

3. Add the tomatoes, olives, chickpeas, salt, and beef. Bring to a simmer and cook, covered, for 10 minutes or until the vegetables are tender. Remove from the heat and stir in the hot sauce. Serve with the couscous and sprinkle with the pistachios.

MAKES 4 SERVINGS

PER SERVING: 403 calories; 13 g total fat; 3 g saturated fat; 46 g carbohydrate; 10 g fiber; 28 g protein; 53 mg cholesterol; 687 mg sodium

NOTE: This recipe is a little high in sodium (you want to aim for no more than 600 to 650 milligrams per meal), so be sure to work this recipe into your daily total of 2,300 milligrams of sodium by selecting recipes for the remaining meals that are around 300 to 400 milligrams each.

12 ounces 95% lean ground beef

½ tablespoon olive oil

1 medium eggplant, peeled and cut into 1" cubes

2 small yellow squash, cut into quarter rounds

4 cloves garlic, smashed

1 teaspoon garam masala

½ teaspoon ground cinnamon

1 tablespoon slivered fresh ginger

1 can (14.5 ounces) diced tomatoes with basil and oregano

½ cup small pitted black olives, halved

½ cup canned chickpeas, rinsed and drained

⅛ teaspoon salt

2 to 3 teaspoons mild hot sauce

2 cups cooked whole wheat couscous

2 tablespoons chopped pistachios

CHAPTER 6 ∘ DINNERS

GROUND BEEF AND PASTA SKILLET DINNER

4 ounces whole grain penne pasta

2 tablespoons olive oil

1 large onion, chopped

2 red bell peppers, chopped

3 cloves garlic, finely minced

1 pound 95% lean ground beef

2 cans (14.5 ounces each) no-salt-added tomatoes

2 cups chopped baby spinach

1 teaspoon dried oregano or Italian seasoning

½ teaspoon salt

2 tablespoons pine nuts, toasted

FOR THE BEST flavor, take the time to let the beef fully brown before incorporating the other ingredients. This is a dish that will easily appeal to diners of all ages.

TOTAL TIME: 50 MINUTES

1. Prepare the pasta according to package directions.

2. Meanwhile, heat the oil in a large skillet over medium heat. Cook the onion, peppers, and garlic, stirring, for 3 minutes. Add the beef and cook, stirring, for 5 minutes, or until browned and no longer pink.

3. Stir in the tomatoes, spinach, oregano, salt, and cooked pasta.

4. Sprinkle the top with pine nuts.

MAKES 4 SERVINGS

PER SERVING: 429 calories; 16 g total fat; 4 g saturated fat; 38 g carbohydrate; 7 g fiber; 33 g protein; 70 mg cholesterol; 429 mg sodium

---

DIET DILEMMA: HANDLING FOOD PUSHERS

Problem: We all have those friends or family members—the ones who say, "Just have one more piece!" or "I'm having dessert, you *have* to eat some too!" These are food pushers—people who try (intentionally or unintentionally) to sabotage your diet.

Solution: If it's a good friend or close family member who's a pusher, try being direct, and explain that you're really committed to losing weight and you want it to work. If the food pusher isn't someone you can refuse (like your boss), take a few small bites, and then put down your fork.

SLOW-COOKED PORK WITH BLACK BEANS

S LOW COOKERS ARE a great way to cook when you are short on time. Simply put the ingredients in the cooker, head out for the day, and when you return, there will be a meal awaiting you.

TOTAL TIME: 7 HOURS

1. Place the pork, tomatoes, garlic, onion, beans, molasses, chili powder, coriander, ¼ teaspoon of the salt, and ½ cup water in a 4- to 6-quart slow cooker. Cover and cook on low for 7 to 9 hours, or on high for 3½ to 4 hours.

2. About 15 minutes before the pork is ready, mash the avocado with the back of a fork in a large bowl. Stir in the lime juice and the remaining ¼ teaspoon salt. Stir in the lettuce and cilantro.

3. Remove the pork from the slow cooker and shred it with a fork. Put the shredded pork back in the slow cooker. Serve the pork in bowls and top with the avocado salad.

MAKES 4 SERVINGS

PER SERVING: 336 calories; 10 g total fat; 2 g saturated fat; 35 g carbohydrate; 10 g fiber; 33 g protein; 78 mg cholesterol; 630 mg sodium

1 pound boneless pork center loin, trimmed

4 tomatoes, chopped

2 cloves garlic, minced

1 onion, chopped

1 can (15.5 ounces) reduced-sodium black beans, rinsed and drained

1 tablespoon molasses

2 teaspoons chili powder

1 teaspoon ground coriander

½ teaspoon salt, divided

1 avocado, skin and pit removed

1 tablespoon fresh lime juice

2 cups shredded romaine lettuce

1 cup chopped cilantro

CHAPTER 6 ○ DINNERS

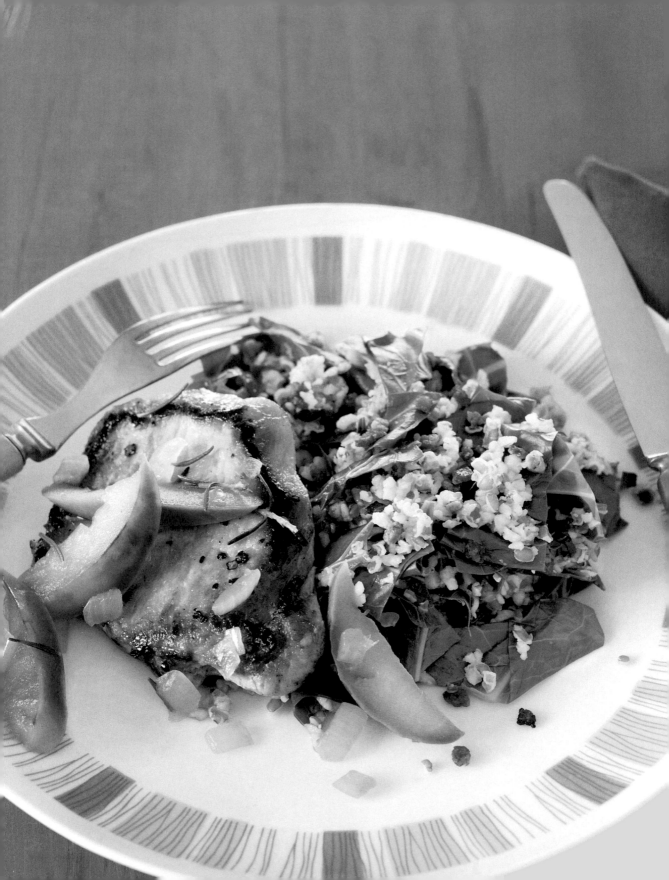

PORK CHOPS WITH APPLES AND COLLARD GREENS

BULGUR IS A great addition to your meals and a great source of fiber. Bulgur or cracked wheat is a toasted, chopped form of the whole wheat berry and a staple in Middle Eastern cooking.

TOTAL TIME: 35 MINUTES

1. Coat a large saucepan with cooking spray and heat it over medium-high heat. Cook the bacon and collard greens, for 2 minutes, stirring often. Add the vinegar, cayenne pepper (if desired), and 2 cups water. Bring to a boil, reduce the heat to low, cover, and simmer for 15 minutes. Stir in the bulgur and ¼ teaspoon of the salt. Remove from the heat. Cover and set aside.

2. Meanwhile, heat 1 tablespoon of the oil in a large skillet over medium heat. Cook the apples, onion, and rosemary, stirring often, for 5 minutes, or until lightly browned. Add 2 tablespoons of water and ¼ teaspoon of the remaining salt; cook for 5 minutes. Transfer to a plate and set aside.

3. Rub the pork chops with the remaining ¼ teaspoon salt and the pepper. Heat the remaining 1 tablespoon oil in the same skillet over medium-high heat. Cook the pork chops, turning once, for 6 minutes, or until lightly browned and a thermometer inserted in the center of a chop registers 160°F and the juices run clear.

4. Divide the collard greens among 4 plates. Top each with a pork chop and the apple mixture.

MAKES 4 SERVINGS

PER SERVING: 406 calories; 13 g total fat; 3 g saturated fat; 42 g carbohydrate; 11 g fiber; 32 g protein; 66 mg cholesterol; 592 mg sodium

1 ounce Canadian bacon, finely chopped

6 cups chopped collard greens

2 tablespoons apple cider vinegar

⅛ to ¼ teaspoon cayenne pepper (optional)

1 cup bulgur (cracked wheat)

¾ teaspoon salt, divided

2 tablespoons olive oil, divided

2 Golden Delicious or Granny Smith apples, cored and thinly sliced

1 onion, finely chopped

1 tablespoon chopped fresh rosemary

4 boneless pork chops (4 ounces each)

¼ teaspoon pepper

CHAPTER 6 • DINNERS

PORK LOIN WITH SUCCOTASH

½ teaspoon ground cinnamon

½ teaspoon ground cumin

¼ teaspoon cocoa powder

1 tablespoon + 1 teaspoon brown sugar, divided

¾ teaspoon salt, divided

3 tablespoons olive oil, divided

1 pound pork tenderloin

2 cups shredded red cabbage

2 tablespoons cider vinegar

1 onion, thinly sliced

2 zucchini or yellow squash, sliced

2 tablespoons fresh chopped thyme or 2 teaspoons dried

1 cup fresh or frozen and thawed lima beans

1 cup fresh or frozen and thawed corn

THE DRY RUB really penetrates the pork and makes this an outstanding dish. If you have time, let the marinating pork rest in the refrigerator for 24 hours before cooking.

TOTAL TIME: 40 MINUTES PLUS MARINATING TIME

1. Blend the cinnamon, cumin, cocoa powder, 1 tablespoon of the brown sugar, ¼ teaspoon of the salt, and 1½ tablespoons of the oil in a food processor until it forms a paste.

2. Place the pork in a roasting pan and rub the mixture over the pork. Marinate at room temperature for 1 hour or refrigerate for up to 24 hours.

3. Preheat the oven to 375°F.

4. Roast the pork for 20 to 25 minutes, or until a thermometer inserted in the center registers 155°F and the juices run clear. Let stand for 10 minutes before slicing.

5. Meanwhile, in a large bowl, combine the cabbage, vinegar, the remaining 1½ tablespoons oil, 1 teaspoon brown sugar, and the remaining ¼ teaspoon of the salt. Cover and chill.

6. Heat a large saucepan coated with cooking spray over medium-high heat. Cook the onion for 3 minutes. Add the squash, thyme, and the remaining ¼ teaspoon salt and cook, stirring, for 5 minutes. Add the lima beans, corn, and 1 cup water and cook for 2 to 5 minutes, or until lima beans are tender. Fresh may take longer than frozen.

7. Divide the pork, succotash, and cabbage salad among 4 plates.

MAKES 4 SERVINGS

PER SERVING: 363 calories; 13 g total fat; 2 g saturated fat; 33 g carbohydrate; 6 g fiber; 30 g protein; 74 mg cholesterol; 542 mg sodium

PORK
SATAY

I F YOU'RE NOT into threading skewers, slice the pork into 1" pieces, pound to ¼" thick, and marinate and grill as directed. The salad can be assembled (but not tossed) and refrigerated up to 2 hours in advance.

TOTAL TIME: 35 MINUTES

1. Cut the pork in half crosswise. Place in the freezer for 15 minutes, to facilitate slicing. Grate 1 teaspoon lime zest; cut the lime into wedges for serving.

2. Bring 4 cups of water to a boil in a medium saucepan. Add the edamame and corn. Cook for 4 minutes, or just until tender. Drain and rinse under cold running water.

3. Slice each piece of pork lengthwise into 4 strips and place in a medium bowl. Add the lime zest and 2 tablespoons of the dressing; toss to coat. Set aside to marinate for 15 minutes. Thread the pork onto four 8" skewers.

4. Preheat a grill or grill pan over medium-high heat. In a large bowl, whisk together the remaining dressing and the honey and vinegar. Add the carrots, corn mixture, cucumber, and cilantro. Toss right before serving and top with the peanuts.

5. Grill the skewers, turning once, for 4 minutes, or until the meat is no longer pink. Serve with the vegetable salad and the lime wedges.

MAKES 2 SERVINGS

PER SERVING: 400 calories; 22 g total fat; 3 g saturated fat; 25 g carbohydrate; 6 g fiber; 28 g protein; 55 mg cholesterol; 393 mg sodium

6 ounces pork tenderloin, (about ½ whole tenderloin)

1 large lime

½ cup frozen shelled edamame

½ cup frozen corn

¼ cup sesame ginger dressing, divided

1 teaspoon honey

2 teaspoons balsamic vinegar

½ cup shredded carrots

½ small cucumber. peeled. seeded, and cut into julienne strips

¼ cup coarsely chopped cilantro

2 tablespoons peanuts

CHAPTER 6 ○ DINNERS

PORK AND PLUM KEBABS

SAUCE

2 cloves garlic, chopped

1 tomato, chopped

1 small onion, chopped

¼ cup balsamic vinegar

1 tablespoon molasses

¼ teaspoon salt

⅛ to ¼ teaspoon cayenne pepper

KEBABS

2 plums, pitted and cut into 6 wedges each

2 onions, cut into 6 wedges each

12 ounces boneless pork loin, cut into 1½" cubes

1 tablespoon chopped fresh oregano

4 tablespoons olive oil, divided

1 tablespoon fresh lemon juice

¼ teaspoon salt

¼ teaspoon black pepper

4 cups chopped romaine lettuce

4 whole grain dinner rolls

THE COOKING INSTRUCTIONS call for a broiler, but the kebabs would also be delicious prepared on an indoor or outdoor grill. Make the sauce ahead and refrigerate for up to 4 days.

TOTAL TIME: 55 MINUTES

TO MAKE THE SAUCE

1. Place the garlic, tomato, onion, vinegar, molasses, salt, and cayenne pepper in a small saucepan. Bring to a boil, reduce the heat to low, and simmer for 25 minutes. Puree in a food processor or blender until smooth; set aside.

TO MAKE THE KEBABS

1. Preheat the broiler.
2. Combine the plums, onions, pork, oregano and 2 tablespoons of the olive oil in a large bowl. Toss to coat well. Thread onto four 12" skewers.
3. Place on the rack of a broiling pan and broil, turning once, for 8 minutes, or until a thermometer inserted in the center registers 155°F and the juices run clear.
3. Whisk together the lemon juice, salt, black pepper and the 2 tablespoons olive oil in a large bowl. Add the lettuce and toss to coat.
4. Divide the pork, plums, and onion among 4 plates. Drizzle with the sauce. Divide the salad and rolls among the plates.

MAKES 4 SERVINGS

PER SERVING: 374 calories; 19 g total fat; 3 g saturated fat; 34 g carbohydrate; 4 g fiber; 24 g protein; 59 mg cholesterol; 555 mg sodium

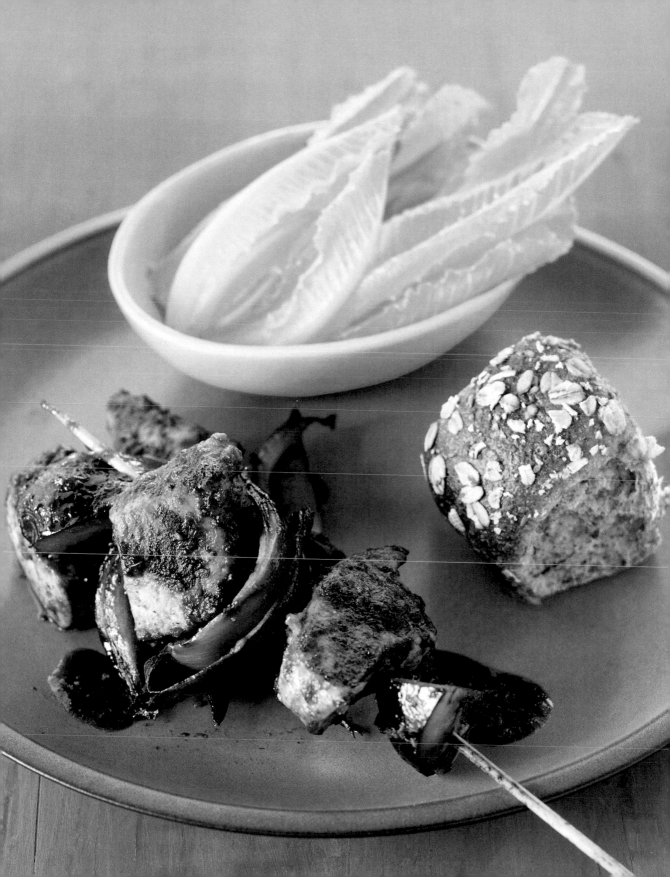

APRICOT-GLAZED PORK SKEWERS

1 cup shelled, frozen edamame

5 scallions, divided

¼ cup apricot spreadable fruit

2 teaspoons Dijon mustard

1½ teaspoons grated fresh ginger, divided

3 tablespoons seasoned rice wine vinegar, divided

¼ teaspoon salt, divided

¼ teaspoon freshly ground pepper, divided

8 ounces pork tenderloin, trimmed and cut into ¾" cubes

1 large red or yellow bell pepper, cut into ¾" pieces

½ large cucumber, seeded and chopped (1 cup)

¼ cup peanuts, chopped

TOSS THIS TASTY cucumber salad with 3 ounces of smoked tofu for a refreshing lunch. If you wish, substitute half or all of the edamame with frozen peas and try diced jicama in place of the cucumber.

TOTAL TIME: 35 MINUTES

1. Preheat a grill or broiler to medium-high. Bring 2 cups of water to a boil in a saucepan. Add the edamame and cook for 5 minutes, or until tender. Drain, rinse under cold water, and set aside. Finely chop 2 scallions; cut the remaining scallions into 1½" lengths.

2. In a medium bowl, whisk together the spreadable fruit, mustard, 1 teaspoon of the ginger, 1½ tablespoons vinegar, half of the chopped scallions, ⅛ teaspoon of the salt, and ⅛ teaspoon of the pepper. Set aside 3 tablespoons of the sauce in a small dish for serving.

3. Alternately thread the pork, bell pepper, and scallion pieces onto four 10" skewers.

4. Grill or broil the skewers for 6 to 8 minutes, turning them once, then brushing with the remaining sauce.

5. Meanwhile, in a medium bowl, combine the cucumber and edamame with the remaining 1½ tablespoons vinegar, ½ teaspoon ginger, chopped scallions, ⅛ teaspoon salt, and ⅛ teaspoon pepper. Serve the pork skewers with the cucumber salad, reserved sauce, and scatter both with the peanuts.

MAKES 2 SERVINGS

PER SERVING: 425 calories; 11 g total fat; 1 g saturated fat; 44 g carbohydrate; 8 g fiber; 38 g protein; 74 mg cholesterol; 695 mg sodium

NOTE: This recipe is a little high in sodium (you want to aim for no more than 600 to 650 milligrams per meal), so be sure to work this recipe into your daily total of 2,300 milligrams of sodium by selecting recipes for your remaining meals that have around 300 to 400 milligrams each.

SALMON WITH WILD RICE SALAD

YOU MAY WANT to wear gloves while shredding the beet to avoid turning your hands bright pink. For variety, baby spinach or arugula works nicely in place of the spinach.

TOTAL TIME: 45 MINUTES

1. Prepare the rice according to package directions.

2. In a large bowl, combine the spinach, celery, beet, vinegar, oil, nuts, pepper, and ½ teaspoon salt. Stir in the hot rice.

3. Heat a large nonstick skillet coated with cooking spray over medium heat. Cook the salmon, turning once, for 6 minutes or until the fish is opaque. Sprinkle with the remaining ¼ teaspoon salt.

4. Divide the fish and salad among 4 plates.

MAKES 4 SERVINGS

PER SERVING: 416 calories; 16 g total fat; 2 g saturated fat; 38 g carbohydrate; 5 g fiber; 30 g protein; 62 mg cholesterol; 575 mg sodium

1 cup wild rice

4 cups chopped spinach

2 ribs celery, sliced

1 beet, shredded

3 tablespoons balsamic vinegar

2 tablespoons olive oil

4 teaspoons pine nuts

¼ teaspoon pepper

¾ teaspoon salt, divided

4 wild salmon fillets (4 ounces each)

CHAPTER 6 ∘ DINNERS

METABOLISM BOOSTER: SEEK OUT SPICE

Spicy food can do more than just set your tongue on fire. Did you know that adding heat can also help you subtract calories? It might do so by speeding up your metabolism and helping you burn more calories. Many spicy foods get their heat from capsaicin, the major hot component of peppers such as jalapeños and cayenne. One study found that people who ate a breakfast containing capsaicin burned 23 percent more calories after the meal than those who ate a nonspiced meal.[1] Spicy foods can also help decrease your calorie consumption: Study participants who ate an appetizer with a hot red-pepper sauce ate significantly fewer calories than people who ate a sauceless appetizer.[2] It's time to turn up the heat!

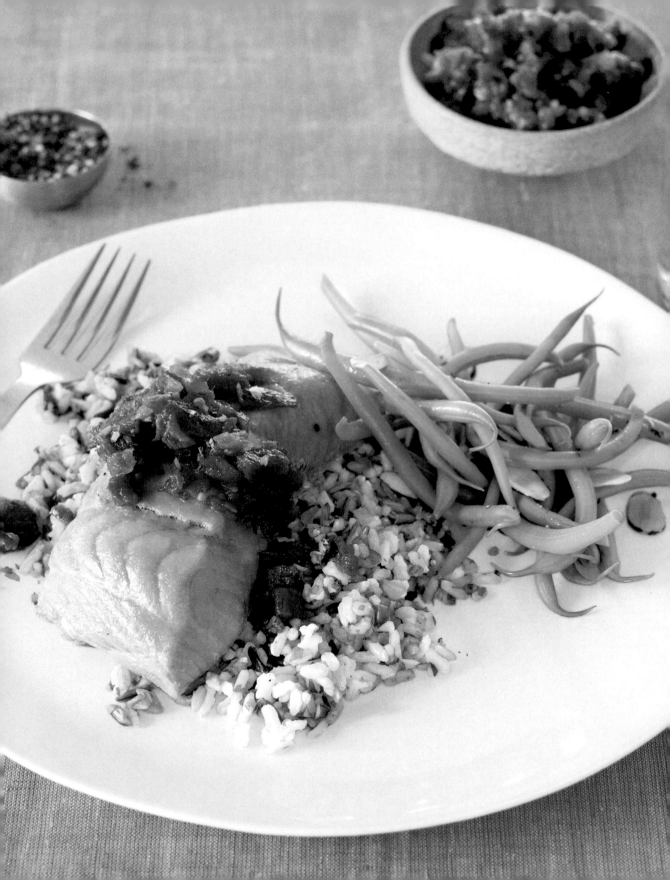

SLOW-ROASTED SALMON WITH TOMATO-GINGER JAM

SLOW ROASTING IS a fail-proof way to avoid overcooking fish, producing perfectly cooked fish every time. This tasty tomato jam will also pair nicely with cooked chicken, pork, or beef. Great for entertaining, you can make the jam ahead and reheat in the microwave just before serving.

TOTAL TIME: 35 MINUTES

1. Preheat the oven to 250°F. Coat a baking sheet with cooking spray.

2. Place the salmon on the baking sheet and sprinkle with the salt and pepper. Bake for 25 minutes, or until just cooked through.

3. Meanwhile, heat 1 teaspoon of the oil in a small saucepan over medium heat. Add the onion and cook for 6 minutes, stirring, until softened. Stir in the tomatoes, honey, vinegar, ginger, and paprika. Bring to a simmer and cook for 8 minutes, or until reduced to a jamlike consistency. Stir in the mint.

4. Toss the green beans, almonds, and the remaining 2 teaspoons olive oil in a large bowl. Divide the salmon, jam, green beans, and rice among 4 large plates.

MAKES 4 SERVINGS

PER SERVING: 432 calories; 16 g total fat; 2 g saturated fat; 43 g carbohydrate; 7 g fiber; 29 g protein; 62 mg cholesterol; 451 mg sodium

4 salmon fillets
    (5 ounces each)

¼ teaspoon salt

¼ teaspoon ground black
    pepper

3 teaspoons olive oil,
    divided

1 small red onion, finely
    chopped

1 can (15 ounces) petite
    diced tomatoes with
    basil and oregano

2 tablespoons honey

2 tablespoons red wine
    vinegar

2 teaspoons grated fresh
    ginger

1 teaspoon smoked paprika

2 teaspoons chopped fresh
    mint

3 cups green beans,
    steamed

6 tablespoons toasted
    sliced almonds

2 cups cooked brown rice

CHAPTER 6 ∘ DINNERS

POACHED SALMON AND BARLEY SALAD

½ cup medium pearled barley

3 tablespoons Dijon mustard

2 tablespoons olive oil

2 teaspoons honey

½ teaspoon salt, divided

4 cups shredded romaine lettuce

2 carrots, shredded

1 bunch parsley, chopped

¼ cup almonds, chopped

½ cup white wine or apple juice

½ onion, finely chopped

1 tablespoon fresh thyme

4 wild salmon fillets (4 ounces each)

1 tablespoon fresh lemon juice

THE BARLEY SALAD for this dish can be made 24 hours in advance and stored in the refrigerator. Poaching is an excellent technique to infuse flavor into the salmon and retain moistness.

TOTAL TIME: 50 MINUTES

1. Prepare the barley according to package directions.

2. In a large bowl, whisk together the mustard, oil, honey, and ¼ teaspoon of the salt. Add the lettuce, carrots, parsley, almonds, and cooked barley. Toss to coat well. Set aside.

3. In a large skillet, combine the wine, onion, thyme, and 2 cups of water. Bring to a boil. Reduce the heat to low and simmer for 5 minutes. Add the fish. Cover and cook for 5 minutes, or until the fish is opaque.

4. Remove the salmon from the cooking liquid and place on 4 plates. Sprinkle with the lemon juice and the remaining ¼ teaspoon salt. Divide the salad among the plates.

MAKES 4 SERVINGS

PER SERVING: 421 calories; 17 g total fat; 2 g saturated fat; 34 g carbohydrate; 7 g fiber; 28 g protein; 62 mg cholesterol; 648 mg sodium

ASIAN SALMON SALAD

"SALMON IS WELL known to be one of the best anti-aging foods available, packed with protein and healthy omega-3 fats. I love it topped with this Asian dressing. This is not just a salad but truly a meal and a once-a-week dish for me."

TOTAL TIME: 15 MINUTES

1. Preheat the broiler.
2. Place the salmon on a rack in a broiler pan. Sprinkle with the salt and pepper. Broil 4″ from the heat for 6 to 8 minutes, or until the fish is opaque.
3. In a large bowl, whisk together the vinegar, soy sauce, sugar, and sesame oil until the sugar dissolves. Whisk in the olive oil until well blended. Add the greens and carrots, and toss to coat.
4. Divide the salad among 4 plates. Sprinkle each with 1 tablespoon of the almonds. Serve each with 1 salmon fillet.

MAKES 4 SERVINGS

PER SERVING: 401 calories; 26 g total fat; 4 g saturated fat; 18 g carbohydrate; 4 g fiber; 26 g protein; 62 mg cholesterol; 531 mg sodium

4 salmon fillets (4 ounces each)

¼ teaspoon salt

¼ teaspoon pepper

3 tablespoons rice wine vinegar

2 tablespoons reduced-sodium soy sauce

2 tablespoons brown sugar

2 teaspoons toasted sesame oil

¼ cup olive oil

2 bags (7 ounces each) mixed greens

3 carrots, shredded

¼ cup sliced almonds, toasted

CHAPTER 6 ∘ DINNERS

MOROCCAN SHRIMP SKEWERS

¾ cup bulgur (cracked wheat)

1 tablespoon ground coriander

2 teaspoons mild smoked paprika

2 teaspoons crushed or ground fennel seed

½ teaspoon salt, divided

½ teaspoon freshly ground black pepper, divided

1¼ pounds large shrimp, peeled and deveined, with tails on

3 medium yellow squash (or mixture of yellow and zucchini), cut into ½" thick half rounds

24 large grape tomatoes

1 pickling cucumber or 1 small cucumber, chopped

½ ripe avocado, chopped

¼ cup chopped parsley

2 tablespoons lemon juice

1 tablespoon olive oil

1 teaspoon lemon zest

Y OU CAN ASSEMBLE these skewers and make the bulgur salad up to 3 hours in advance. Coating wooden skewers with cooking spray prevents the likelihood of burning the wood.

TOTAL TIME: 35 MINUTES

1. Bring 2 cups of water to a boil in a small saucepan. Add the bulgur. Remove from the heat, cover, and let stand for 40 to 60 minutes, or until tender-firm. Drain any excess water.

2. Meanwhile, in a small bowl, combine the coriander, paprika, fennel seed, ¼ teaspoon of the salt, and ¼ teaspoon of the pepper. Alternately skewer the shrimp, squash, and tomatoes onto twelve 12" wooden skewers.

3. Coat the prepared skewers with cooking spray. Sprinkle the spice mixture evenly over both sides of the skewers.

4. Preheat the grill or heat a grill pan over medium heat. Grill the skewers for 8 minutes, turning once, or until the shrimp are opaque and the vegetables are tender.

5. In a large bowl, combine the bulgur, cucumber, avocado, parsley, lemon juice, oil, lemon zest, the remaining ¼ teaspoon salt, and ¼ teaspoon pepper. Toss to coat well.

6. Divide the skewers and salad among 4 plates.

MAKES 4 SERVINGS

PER SERVING: 380 calories; 12 g total fat; 2 g saturated fat; 35 g carbohydrate; 11 g fiber; 36 g protein; 215 mg cholesterol; 530 mg sodium

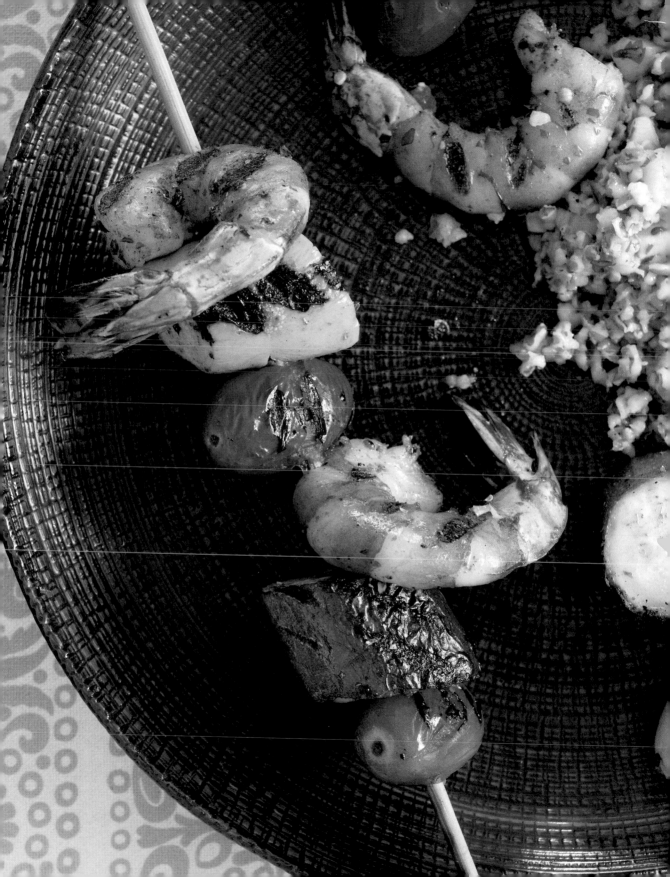

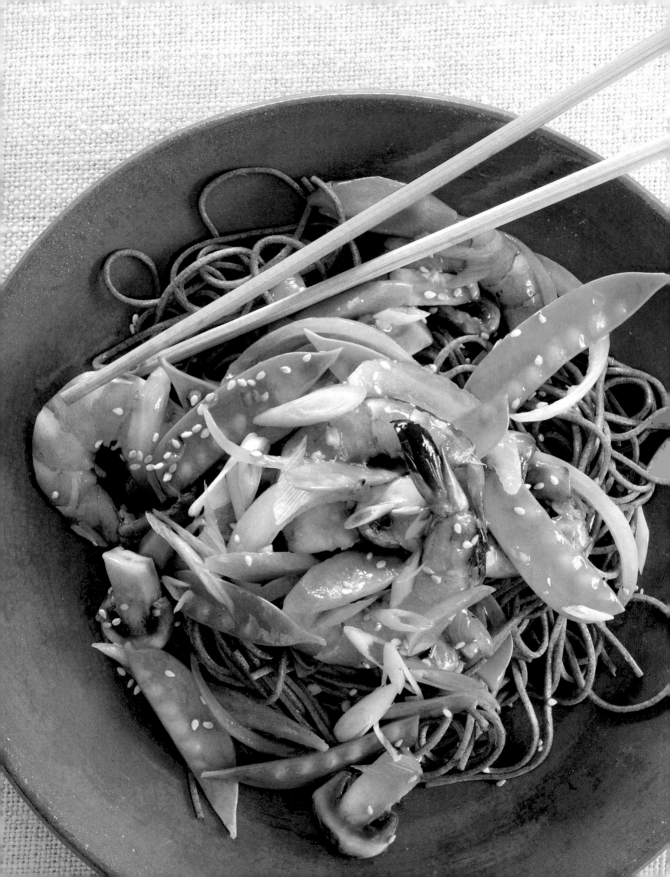

STIR-FRIED SHRIMP ON NOODLES

To MINIMIZE CLEANUP, use the same skillet to cook the vegetables and the shrimp, without washing in between. If you want to make this dinner ahead, prepare all of the vegetables and the noodles up to 24 hours in advance and store them in the refrigerator.

TOTAL TIME: 30 MINUTES

1. Prepare the noodles according to package directions.

2. Whisk together the cornstarch and ½ cup of water in a small bowl. Stir in the soy sauce, vinegar, and sesame oil. Set aside.

3. Heat the canola oil in a large nonstick skillet or wok over medium-high heat. Cook the garlic, onion, and ginger, stirring, for 2 minutes or until lightly browned.

4. Add the mushrooms, snow peas, and carrots and cook, stirring, for 5 minutes or until browned. Remove to a plate.

5. Coat the same skillet or wok, with cooking spray and heat it over medium-high heat. Cook the shrimp, stirring for 3 minutes, or until opaque. Stir the cornstarch mixture and add it to the skillet with the vegetables. Cook, stirring constantly, for 2 minutes, or until thickened.

6. Divide the noodles and shrimp mixture among 4 plates. Sprinkle with the scallions and sesame seeds.

MAKES 4 SERVINGS

PER SERVING: 389 calories; 14 g total fat; 2 g saturated fat; 41 g carbohydrate; 7 g fiber; 28 g protein; 129 mg cholesterol; 453 mg sodium

4 ounces soba (buckwheat) noodles

2 teaspoons cornstarch

2 tablespoons reduced-sodium soy sauce

2 tablespoons rice wine vinegar

1 tablespoon toasted sesame oil

1 tablespoon canola oil

4 cloves garlic, minced

1 onion, sliced

1 tablespoon grated fresh ginger

½ pound white mushrooms, sliced

¼ pound snow peas, trimmed

2 carrots, diagonally sliced

12 ounces peeled and deveined shrimp

2 scallions, thinly sliced

1 tablespoon sesame seeds

SHRIMP MINESTRONE

1 cup brown rice elbow pasta

2 tablespoons olive oil

1 onion, chopped

1 package (32 ounces) low-sodium vegetable broth

8 ounces green beans, cut in half

4 tomatoes, chopped

2 carrots, chopped

1 tablespoon chopped fresh oregano

1 tablespoon chopped fresh thyme

12 ounces shrimp, peeled and deveined

¼ teaspoon pepper

¼ cup grated Parmesan cheese

THIS HEARTY SOUP is good year-round. The fresh herbs bring intensity and lightness to the dish. For optimum texture and flavor, take care not to overcook the shrimp.

TOTAL TIME: 30 MINUTES

1. Prepare the pasta according to package directions.

2. Meanwhile, heat the oil in a large saucepan over medium heat. Cook the onion, stirring, for 5 minutes. Add the broth, green beans, tomatoes, carrots, oregano, thyme, and 2 cups of water.

3. Bring to a boil and reduce the heat to low. Simmer for 15 minutes. Add the shrimp, pasta, and pepper.

4. Return to a simmer and cook for 3 minutes, or until the shrimp are opaque. Divide among 4 bowls and top each with 1 tablespoon of the cheese.

MAKES 4 SERVINGS

PER SERVING: 389 calories; 11 g total fat; 2 g saturated fat; 40 g carbohydrate; 6 g fiber; 30 g protein; 177 mg cholesterol; 413 mg sodium

ROASTED COD WITH BROCCOLI AND MASHED POTATOES

ROASTING BRINGS OUT the natural sweetness of vegetables. As they brown, the veggies caramelize creating a pleasant flavor that masks any bitterness. Coating the vegetables with cooking spray is a low-fat way to roast vegetables.

TOTAL TIME: 30 MINUTES

1. Preheat the oven to 400°F. Lightly coat 2 rimmed baking sheets with cooking spray.

2. Place the potatoes in a medium saucepan and cover with water. Bring to a boil over high heat. Cook for 15 minutes, or until the potatoes are fork-tender. Drain and return to the pan. Mash the potatoes with the oil, basil, and ½ teaspoon of the salt. Keep them warm.

3. Meanwhile, spread the broccoli and garlic over 1½ of the baking sheets (leaving room to roast the cod), and lightly coat them with cooking spray. Roast in the oven for a total of 20 minutes, or until tender and lightly browned on the edges. After 10 minutes, carefully place the cod on the baking pan, and sprinkle it with the remaining ¼ teaspoon salt. Roast for 5 to 7 minutes or until the fish flakes easily and the vegetables are tender-crisp. Place the cod on a platter and the vegetables in a bowl. Toss the vegetables with the vinegar.

4. Divide the cod, potatoes, and vegetables among 4 plates.

MAKES 4 SERVINGS

PER SERVING: 364 calories; 15 g total fat; 2 g saturated fat; 32 g carbohydrate; 6 g fiber; 27 g protein; 42 mg cholesterol; 577 mg sodium

1 pound Yukon gold or red potatoes, peeled and cut into 1" cubes

¼ cup olive oil

¼ cup chopped fresh basil

¾ teaspoon salt, divided

1 head broccoli, cut into florets

4 cloves garlic, minced

1 pound wild cod, cut into 4 portions

2 tablespoons balsamic vinegar

CHAPTER 6 ∘ DINNERS

GRILLED WHITEFISH WITH EDAMAME PESTO

½ cup cooked edamame

½ cup fresh basil leaves

¼ cup parsley leaves

¼ cup Parmesan cheese

¼ cup walnuts

1½ tablespoons olive oil

½ teaspoon salt, divided

¼ teaspoon freshly ground pepper, divided

1¼ pounds cod, scrod, or other firm whitefish fillet, cut into 4 pieces

1 large red sweet onion, cut into wedges

1 pound asparagus, trimmed

2 small ears corn, halved

MAKE THIS PESTO up to 6 hours in advance and cover it with plastic pressed onto the surface to prevent discoloration. This versatile pesto is great served with steak, chicken, or pork. If you find yourself with leftovers, stir a few tablespoons into a mixture of ¼ cup fat-free plain Greek-style yogurt and ¼ light sour cream. It makes a tasty dip.

TOTAL TIME: 30 MINUTES

1. In a food processor or blender, combine the edamame, basil, parsley, cheese, walnuts, oil, ¼ teaspoon of the salt, ⅛ teaspoon of the pepper, and ⅓ cup of water until smooth. Place in a dish and cover the surface of the pesto with plastic.

2. Preheat the grill or heat a grill pan coated with cooking spray over medium-high heat. Season the fish with the remaining ¼ teaspoon salt and the remaining ⅛ teaspoon pepper and set aside.

3. Grill the onion for 10 minutes, turning once. Grill the asparagus and corn for 6 minutes, turning occasionally. Remove to a serving plate.

4. Reduce the heat to medium. Grill the fish, turning once, for 4 to 6 minutes, or until the fish flakes easily.

5. Divide the fish, onion, asparagus, and corn among 4 plates. Drizzle each with one-quarter of the pesto.

MAKES 4 SERVINGS

PER SERVING: 328 calories; 14 g total fat; 2 g saturated fat; 18 g carbohydrate; 5 g fiber; 35 g protein; 65 mg cholesterol; 485 mg sodium

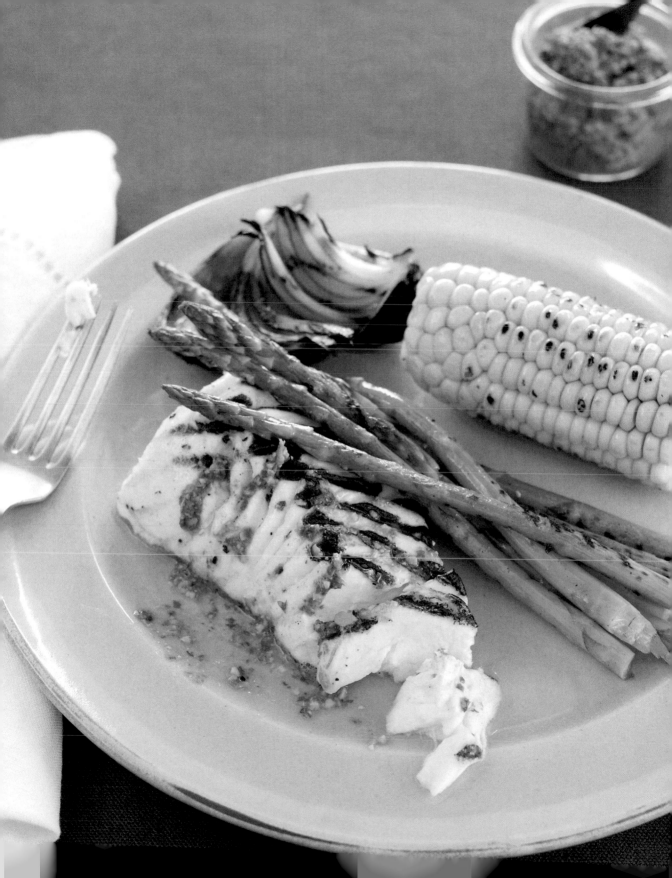

CATFISH PUTTANESCA

½ sweet onion, chopped

1 clove garlic, chopped

½ teaspoon Italian seasoning

1 can (14.5 ounces) no-salt-added diced tomatoes

3 anchovies, chopped

12 kalamata olives, chopped

3 tablespoons chopped parsley

1¼ cups whole wheat panko bread crumbs

2 egg whites

4 catfish or tilapia fillets (1¼ pounds)

¾ teaspoon crab-boil seasoning

1¼ pounds broccolini, trimmed

PANKO BREAD CRUMBS are made in different degrees of coarseness. If they appear too coarse, place them in a food processor and grind them until they're fine, or put them in a bag and press with a rolling pin.

TOTAL TIME: 45 MINUTES

1. Preheat the oven to 425°F. Place a rack on top of a rimmed baking sheet.

2. Coat a medium saucepan with cooking spray and heat it over medium heat. Cook the onion for 6 minutes, or until softened. Stir in the garlic and Italian seasoning and cook for 1 minute. Add the tomatoes, anchovies, and olives. Bring to a simmer and cook for 5 minutes, or until reduced slightly. Stir in the parsley.

3. Meanwhile, place the bread crumbs on a plate. Beat the egg whites in a shallow bowl or pie plate until just frothy. Pat the fish dry with paper towels. Sprinkle both sides of the fillets with the seasoning, rubbing it into the flesh. Dip the fillets in the egg whites and then the crumb mixture, pressing on crumbs to adhere. Coat both sides of the breaded fish with cooking spray and place the fish on the rack in the pan. Bake for 12 to 15 minutes, or until it's golden brown and the fish flakes easily.

4. Place a steamer basket in a medium saucepan filled with 2" of simmering water. Add the broccolini, cover, and steam for 5 minutes, or until tender-crisp.

5. Divide the fish and broccolini among 4 plates.

MAKES 4 SERVINGS

PER SERVING: 421 calories; 15 g total fat; 3 g saturated fat; 36 g carbohydrate; 6 g fiber; 35 g protein; 69 mg cholesterol; 549 mg sodium

FLOUNDER WITH CURRIED VEGETABLES

THIS DELICATE FISH is an excellent companion to the richly flavored curry. Cod, scrod, or tilapia are good substitutes for the flounder. Take care not to overcook the peas and the flounder.

TOTAL TIME: 25 MINUTES

1. Heat the oil in a Dutch oven or stockpot over medium heat. Cook the onion, garlic, and ginger, stirring, for 5 minutes. Add the cauliflower, cabbage, okra, cumin, cinnamon, turmeric, salt, cayenne, and 4 cups of water. Bring to a boil. Reduce the heat to low and simmer for 10 minutes, or until the cauliflower is tender.

2. Stir in the peas. Gently stir in the flounder. Cover and simmer for 3 minutes, or until the fish flakes easily.

3. Serve with the yogurt.

MAKES 4 SERVINGS

PER SERVING: 419 calories; 13 g total fat; 1 g saturated fat; 33 g carbohydrate; 12 g fiber; 45 g protein; 82 mg cholesterol; 597 mg sodium

3 tablespoons canola oil

1 onion, sliced

2 cloves garlic, minced

2 teaspoons chopped fresh ginger

1 head cauliflower, chopped

2 cups chopped cabbage

2 cups chopped fresh okra, or ½ bag (16 ounces) frozen

2 teaspoons ground cumin

½ teaspoon ground cinnamon

½ teaspoon ground turmeric

½ teaspoon salt

⅛ to ¼ teaspoon cayenne pepper

2 cups peas, fresh or frozen and thawed

1½ pounds flounder fillets, cut into 2" chunks

½ cup fat-free plain Greek-style yogurt

CARIBBEAN FLOUNDER FILLETS

2 cups quick-cooking brown rice

1 cup reduced-sodium vegetable broth

1 yellow bell pepper, cut into thin strips

8 scallions, sliced on the diagonal into 1" pieces

4 slices lime

3 tablespoons minced fresh cilantro

¼ teaspoon curry powder

4 flounder fillets (about 6 ounces each)

FEEL FREE TO change the bell pepper in this recipe to the red or green, as desired. For a very coloful dish, use half of a red and half of a yellow pepper. You can substitute tilapia or cod for the flounder as well.

TOTAL TIME: 15 MINUTES

1. Prepare rice according to package directions.

2. Meanwhile, in a large nonstick skillet, combine the broth, pepper, scallions, lime, cilantro, and curry powder. Cover and bring to a simmer over medium-high heat.

3. Carefully add the fish. Reduce the heat to medium-low, cover, and gently simmer for 5 to 6 minutes, or until the fish flakes easily. Discard the lime slices.

4. Remove the fish with a slotted spoon and place on 4 plates. Divide the rice and pepper-scallion sauce among the plates.

MAKES 4 SERVINGS

PER SERVING: 310 calories; 3 g total fat; 0 g saturated fat; 38 g carbohydrate; 3 g fiber; 34g protein; 103 mg cholesterol; 224 mg sodium

ARUGULA PESTO PATTIES

THE PATTIES CAN be made ahead and stored tightly wrapped for up to 24 hours before cooking. Leftover brown rice works well but if you do not have any, cook ¾ cup of brown rice (either regular or a quick cooking variety) to yield 2 cups.

TOTAL TIME: 20 MINUTES

1. Remove the tofu from its package and drain in a colander in the sink. Place a flat plate weighted down with a heavy can of vegetables on top of the tofu in the colander for 15 minutes to drain.

2. Preheat the oven to 400°F. Coat a large rimmed baking sheet with cooking spray.

3. Puree the arugula, walnuts, garlic, oil, ⅛ teaspoon salt, and pepper in a food processor for 1 minute or until smooth. Set aside in a small bowl.

4. Puree the tofu in the same food processor for 1 minute or until chopped. Add the rice, half of the onion, oregano, ½ teaspoon of the salt, and 2 tablespoons of the arugula pesto. Puree for 1 minute. Form the mixture into 8 patties.

5. Combine the green beans, cabbage, and the remaining half of a chopped onion on the rimmed baking sheet. Coat with cooking spray and sprinkle with the remaining ⅛ teaspoon salt. Roast for 10 minutes or until the vegetables are lightly browned.

6. Coat a large skillet with cooking spray and cook the patties over medium-high heat, turning once, for 8 minutes or until browned.

7. Place 2 patties on each of 4 plates, with arugula puree, and arrange the vegetables on the side.

MAKES 4 SERVINGS

PER SERVING: 321 calories; 13 g total fat; 1 g saturated fat; 42 g carbohydrate; 9 g fiber; 16 g protein; 0 mg cholesterol; 501 mg sodium

---

1 package (12 ounces drained weight) low-fat extra-firm tofu

4 cups fresh arugula

⅓ cup chopped walnuts

2 cloves garlic, peeled and halved

1 tablespoon olive oil

¾ teaspoon salt, divided

⅛ teaspoon pepper

2 cups cooked brown rice

1 small onion, chopped and divided

1 tablespoon fresh oregano

1 pound green beans

4 cups sliced red cabbage

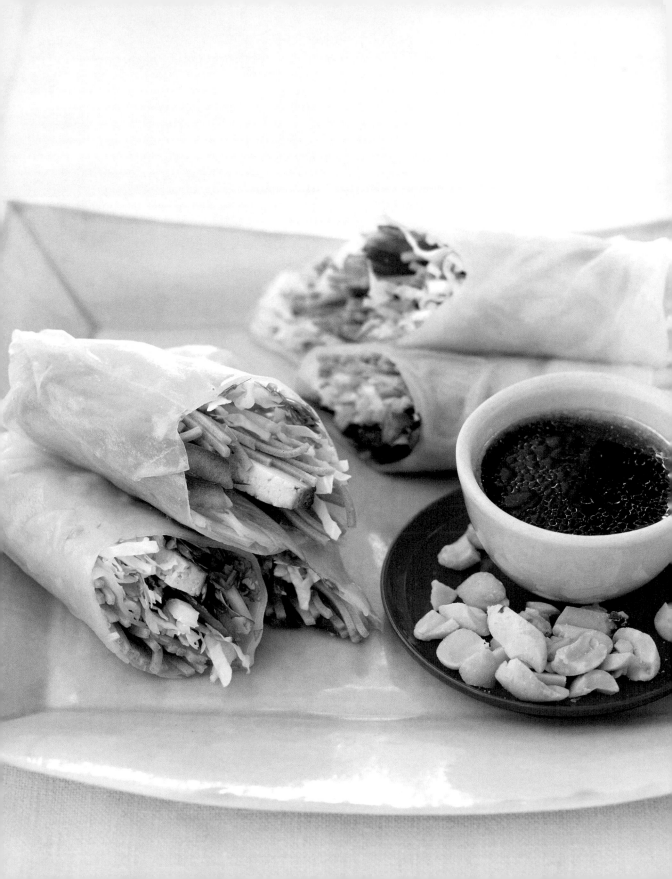

SUMMER ROLLS WITH MARINATED TOFU

ONCE YOU GET the knack of making these, they will go rather quickly. Don't worry if you have a tear in a wrapper—once they are rolled, simply break off a piece of another wrapper, reconstitute it in water, and place over the tear to patch. These tasty rolls can be made ahead and chilled for up to 6 hours.

TOTAL TIME: 45 MINUTES

1. To prepare the sauce, combine the chili sauce, vinegar, soy sauce, ginger, sesame oil, and water in a small dish. Set aside.

2. Cook the noodles according to package directions. Drain well. Place the cabbage, bell pepper, tofu, and noodles on a board for assembling. Toss together the cilantro, mint, and scallions in a medium bowl.

3. Fill a pie plate two-thirds full with room-temperature water. Working with 4 wrappers at a time, dip the rice paper in the water then set on a work surface. Divide ½ cup of the noodles between the wrappers, arranging in a line down the center of each wrapper. Divide ¼ cup each of the cabbage and peppers between the wrappers, 3 tablespoons cilantro mixture, and a few strips of tofu onto the noodles.

4. Fold the 2 sides of the rice paper over the filling, then fold the bottom end over the filling, envelope-style. Roll up tightly, sealing the last side with a little water.

5. Place on a large serving plate or board and cover with damp towels. Repeat with the remaining ingredients. To serve, cut the rolls in half and serve with the sauce and the nuts (if desired).

MAKES 4 SERVINGS

PER SERVING: 396 calories; 12 g total fat; 2 g saturated fat; 47 g carbohydrate; 3 g fiber; 27 g protein; 0 mg cholesterol; 697 mg sodium

NOTE: This recipe is a little high in sodium (you want to aim for no more than 600 to 650 milligrams per meal), so be sure to work this recipe into your daily total of 2,300 milligrams of sodium by selecting recipes for the remaining meals that are around 300 to 400 milligrams each.

DIPPING SAUCE

2 tablespoons sweet Asian chili sauce

1 tablespoon rice or white wine vinegar

1½ teaspoons reduced-sodium soy sauce

½ teaspoon grated fresh ginger

1½ teaspoons toasted sesame oil

1 tablespoon water

SUMMER ROLLS

3 ounces buckwheat noodles

1½ cups thinly sliced Napa cabbage

1 red bell pepper, thinly sliced into 2" pieces

12 ounces teriyaki marinated tofu, cut into strips

½ cup chopped cilantro leaves

⅓ cup mint or basil leaves, coarsely chopped

2 scallions, sliced

12 round rice paper wrappers (8" diameter)

2 tablespoons unsalted roasted peanuts, chopped (optional)

EDAMAME AND SOBA SALAD

4 ounces soba (buckwheat) noodles

⅔ cup frozen shelled edamame

¼ cup freshly squeezed orange juice

¼ cup tahini (sesame paste)

1 tablespoon toasted sesame oil

1 tablespoon white vinegar

2 teaspoons soy sauce

1 package (12 ounces drained weight) firm tofu, drained and cubed

2 cups bean sprouts

1 large cucumber, thinly sliced

4 cups baby spinach

¼ to ½ teaspoon red pepper flakes

WHEN SELECTING SOBA noodles, read all the nutritional labels before choosing, as some are much higher in sodium than others. Also, choose the one with the most buckwheat, preferably 100%.

TOTAL TIME: 20 MINUTES

1. Prepare the noodles according to package directions, adding the edamame after 1 minute. Drain well.

2. Whisk together the orange juice, tahini, oil, vinegar, and soy sauce in a large bowl. Add the noodles and edamame, tofu, bean sprouts, cucumber, and spinach. Toss to coat well. Sprinkle with the red pepper flakes.

MAKES 4 SERVINGS

PER SERVING: 416 calories; 20 g total fat; 3 g saturated fat; 41 g carbohydrate; 7 g fiber; 26 g protein; 0 mg cholesterol; 513 mg sodium

NOTE: This recipe is a little high in sodium (you want to aim for no more than 600 to 650 milligrams per meal), so be sure to work this recipe into your daily total of 2,300 milligrams of sodium by selecting recipes for the remaining meals that are around 300 to 400 milligrams each.

THAI NOODLE BOWL

CHANGE UP THIS MEAL BY SIMPLY SUBSTITUTING COOKED CHICKEN OR SHRIMP FOR ALL OR PART OF THE TOFU, WHOLE WHEAT OR RICE NOODLES FOR THE SOBA, AND YOUR FAVORITE VEGETABLES FOR THE PEPPER AND MUSHROOMS.

TOTAL TIME: 30 MINUTES

1. Grate the zest of the lime, then juice 2 tablespoons of lime juice and set aside. Bring a large saucepan of water to a boil. Add the noodles and cook 3 minutes or until almost tender. Drain and rinse in a colander; set aside.

2. Heat the broth, coconut milk, honey, curry powder, fish sauce, and 2 cups water to boiling over medium heat in a large saucepan. Add the mushrooms and pepper. Reduce the heat to low and simmer for 2 minutes.

3. Stir in the noodles, snow peas, scallions, tofu, ginger, and lime zest and simmer for 2 minutes. Remove from the heat and stir in the lime juice. Ladle into 4 bowls and sprinkle with the cilantro.

MAKES 4 SERVINGS

PER SERVING: 330 calories; 12 g total fat; 4 g saturated fat; 40 g carbohydrate; 5 g fiber; 22 g protein; 0 mg cholesterol; 434 mg sodium.

1 lime

4 ounces soba (buckwheat) noodles

1 can (14½ ounces) reduced-sodium vegetable broth

1 cup light unsweetened coconut milk, stirred well

2 teaspoons honey

1 teaspoon curry powder

1½ teaspoons lower-sodium fish sauce

1 package (8 ounces) sliced mushrooms

1 red bell pepper, thinly sliced into 2" strips

4 ounces snow peas, halved diagonally

2 scallions, sliced

1 package (12 ounces drained weight) firm tofu, drained and cut into ½" pieces

2 teaspoons grated fresh ginger

½ cup chopped fresh cilantro

LENTIL AND VEGETABLE STEW

2 tablespoons olive oil

1 onion, chopped

2 cloves garlic, minced

12 ounces frozen vegetarian sausage, defrosted and chopped

1 cup lentils

1 carrot, sliced

1 turnip, chopped

½ small rutabaga, chopped

4 cups chopped turnip greens

3 cups low-sodium vegetable broth

1 tablespoons reduced-sodium soy sauce

ROOT VEGETABLES AND lentils are delicious in this hearty stew, making a complete and satisfying meal. When you're pressed for time, prepare the stew ahead and store in the refrigerator for up to 3 days or freeze for up to 3 months.

TOTAL TIME: 1 HOUR

1. Heat the oil in a Dutch oven or stockpot over medium heat.

2. Cook the onion and garlic, stirring often, for 3 minutes. Add the sausage and cook, continuing to stir, for 5 minutes or until well browned.

3. Add the lentils, carrot, turnip, rutabaga, turnip greens, broth, and 3 cups of water. Bring to a boil, reduce the heat to low, cover, and simmer for 45 minutes. Remove from the heat and stir in the soy sauce and salt and black pepper to taste

MAKES 4 SERVINGS

PER SERVING: 415 calories; 8 g total fat; 1 g saturated fat; 58 g carbohydrate; 21 g fiber; 28 g protein; 0 mg cholesterol; 751 mg sodium

NOTE: This recipe is a little high in sodium (you want to aim for no more than 600 to 650 milligrams per meal), so be sure to work this recipe into your daily total of 2,300 milligrams of sodium by selecting recipes for the remaining meals that are around 300 to 400 milligrams each.

TABBOULEH-STUFFED PORTOBELLOS

I F THERE'S ONLY two for dinner, convert this into a double-duty meal. Serve two portobellos for dinner; chop the remaining portobellos, toss with the cracked wheat salad, and spoon over baby arugula for the next day's lunch.

TOTAL TIME: 35 MINUTES

1. Bring 2 cups water to a boil in a small saucepan. Add the bulgur, place the tomatoes on top, cover, and let stand for 40 to 60 minutes or until the bulgur is tender-firm. Drain the bulgur and place in a large bowl. Chop the tomatoes and add to the bowl. (Can be refrigerated for up to 2 days in advance.)

2. Heat a large nonstick skillet coated with cooking spray over medium heat. Cook the zucchini, stirring, for 5 minutes. Add the scallions and carrot and cook for 2 minutes or until just tender. Cool for 10 minutes and add to the bowl with the bulgur and tomatoes.

3. Preheat a grill or grill pan on medium-high heat. Grill the portobellos, rounded-side up, for 4 minutes. Turn and brush with 2 tablespoons pesto. Grill for 4 minutes or until tender. Grill the sausages for 3 to 4 minutes, turning occasionally.

4. Add the lemon juice, mint, pepper, and the remaining 2 tablespoons pesto to the bulgur. Toss to coat well.

5. Place 1 mushroom on each of 4 plates. Top with the bulgur salad. Serve with the sausages.

MAKES 4 SERVINGS

PER SERVING: 326 calories; 6 g total fat; 1 g saturated fat; 48 g carbohydrate; 11 g fiber;
Note: This recipe is a little high in sodium (you want to aim for no more than 600 to 650 mg per meal) so be sure to work this recipe into your daily total of 2,300 mg of sodium by selecting recipes for the remaining meals that are around 300 to 400 mg each.

¾ cup bulgur (cracked wheat)

¼ cup sun-dried tomatoes

2 cups chopped zucchini

2 scallions, chopped

1 cup shredded carrot

4 portobello mushrooms, stems removed

4 tablespoons prepared reduced-fat basil pesto

12 ounces sausage veggie patties, frozen and thawed

2 tablespoons lemon juice

1 tablespoon chopped fresh mint (optional)

¼ teaspoon freshly ground pepper

CHAPTER 6 ◦ DINNERS

EGGPLANT PARMESAN

3 cans (8 ounces each) low-sodium tomato sauce

½ cup refrigerated reduced-fat basil pesto

4 egg whites, beaten

1 cup whole wheat panko bread crumbs

1 medium eggplant (1½ pounds), peeled and cut into ¼" slices

1 package (12 ounces drained weight) firm silken low-fat tofu, drained and patted dry, cut into ¼" slices

¾ cup shredded low-fat Italian cheese blend

⅓ cup grated Parmesan cheese

BAKING EGGPLANT SAVES time and trims calories by reducing the amount of oil used. If you like, make this up to 2 days in advance and reheat at 350°F for 20 to 25 minutes. Serve leftovers in a sandwich, for a tasty treat.

TOTAL TIME: 1¼ HOURS

1. Preheat the oven to 400°F. Coat 2 large baking sheets with olive oil spray. Coat a 9" × 9" baking dish with cooking spray. Combine the tomato sauce and pesto in a medium bowl. Set aside.

2. Beat the egg whites in a shallow dish until foamy. Place the bread crumbs on a sheet of wax paper. Dip the eggplant and tofu slices in the egg whites, then in the crumbs, pressing to coat.

3. Arrange the eggplant and tofu on the baking sheets and coat with cooking spray. Bake for 30 minutes or until golden and tender, turning once and reversing the pans from top to bottom oven rack.

4. Spread ¼ cup of the sauce on the bottom of the baking dish. Arrange the eggplant slices on top. Spoon on half of the remaining sauce and sprinkle on half of the cheeses. Arrange the tofu slices on top. Spoon on the remaining sauce and sprinkle with the remaining cheeses.

5. Bake for 30 minutes or until heated through and the cheese is golden.

MAKES 4 SERVINGS

PER SERVING: 399 calories; 16 g total fat; 6 g saturated fat; 38 g carbohydrate; 9 g fiber; 27 g protein; 25 mg cholesterol; 707 mg sodium

NOTE: This recipe is a little high in sodium (you want to aim for no more than 600 to 650 milligrams per meal), so be sure to work this recipe into your daily total of 2,300 milligrams of sodium by selecting recipes for the remaining meals that are around 300 to 400 milligrams each.

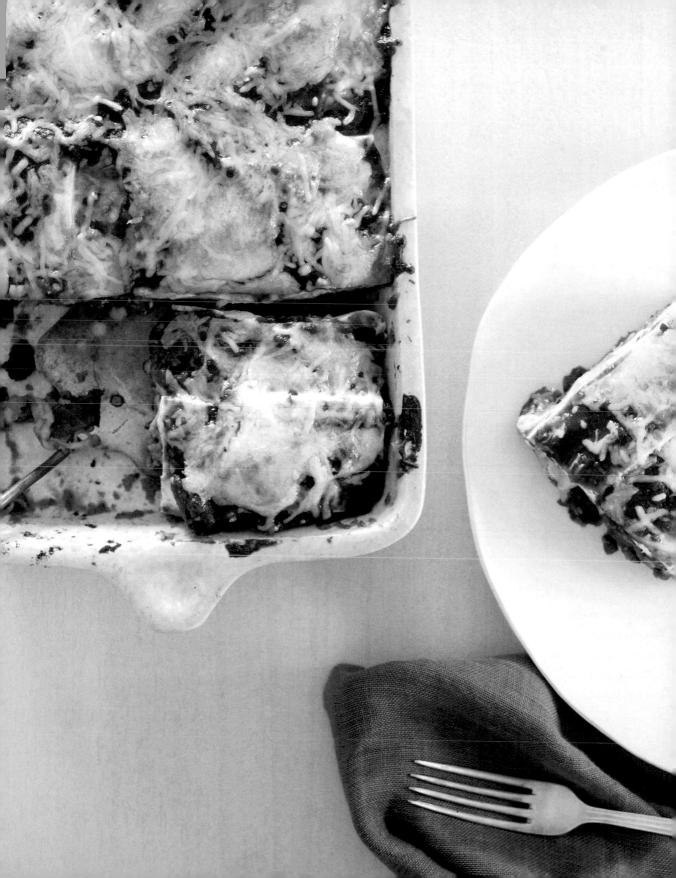

QUINOA CHILI

1 onion, chopped

1 carrot, sliced

½ cup quinoa

1 cup red kidney beans, rinsed and drained

1 package (12 ounces drained weight) firm tofu, drained and cut into cubes

2 tomatoes, chopped

1 tablespoon chili powder

2 teaspoons cocoa powder

¼ to ½ teaspoon cayenne

1 medium avocado, halved, pitted, and peeled

1 tablespoon finely chopped scallion

¼ cup chopped cilantro

2 tablespoons freshly squeezed lime juice

¼ teaspoon salt

WHETHER YOU PREFER your chili mild or spicy, simply adjust the amount of cayenne that you use to suit your taste. The avocado has a nice cooling effect next to the robust full-flavored chili.

TOTAL TIME: 30 MINUTES

1. Heat large saucepot coated with cooking spray over medium heat. Cook the onion and carrot for 5 minutes or until lightly browned.

2. Add the quinoa, beans, tofu, tomatoes, chili powder, cocoa powder, cayenne, and 3 cups of water. Bring to a boil. Reduce the heat to low, cover, and simmer for 20 minutes or until the quinoa is cooked through.

3. Meanwhile, mash the avocado with the scallion, cilantro, lime juice, and the salt in a small bowl.

4. Divide the chili among 4 bowls and top with one-quarter of the avocado mixture.

MAKES 4 SERVINGS

PER SERVING: 363 calories; 15 g total fat; 2 g saturated fat; 39 g carbohydrate; 10 g fiber; 23 g protein; 0 mg cholesterol; 304 mg sodium

MEATLESS SLOPPY JOES

THIS MEATLESS FILLING is served on small whole wheat buns. Flavorful on its own, try this filling in steamed, hollowed-out vegetables such as zucchini, summer squash, or baby eggplant.

TOTAL TIME: 20 MINUTES

1. Heat the oil in a medium nonstick skillet over medium heat. Cook the pepper and onion, stirring occasionally, for 6 minutes or until softened. Add the tempeh and cook, stirring, for 6 minutes or until browned.

2. Add the tomato sauce, honey, vinegar, tamari, and pepper sauce. Bring to a simmer and cook for 4 to 6 minutes, or until sauce has reduced and thickened.

3. Meanwhile, combine the lettuce and carrot in a medium bowl. Toss with the dressing.

4. Place 1 roll on each of 2 plates. Divide the sloppy Joe mixture onto the rolls and serve with the salad.

MAKES 2 SERVINGS

PER SERVING: 411 calories; 6 g total fat; 2 g saturated fat; 70 g carbohydrate; 13 g fiber; 23 g protein; 0 mg cholesterol; 534 mg sodium

1½ teaspoons olive oil

1 green bell pepper, finely chopped

1 medium onion, finely chopped

5 ounces soy tempeh, crumbled

1 can (8 ounces) no-salt-added tomato sauce

3 tablespoons honey

2 teaspoons balsamic vinegar

1 teaspoon reduced-sodium tamari or soy sauce

¼ to ½ teaspoon smoky hot-pepper sauce

3 cups romaine lettuce

1 carrot, shredded

2 tablespoons fat-free ranch dressing

2 whole wheat hamburger rolls

10 quick and easy dinner recipes

dinnertime can be one of the most hectic times of the day. The busiest days are the ones where slipups are most common. Being prepared is necessary if you want to stay on track, regardless of what else is happening. Storing up on certain ingredients—like boneless, skinless chicken breasts, frozen fish, pork cutlets or tenderloins, tofu, and steaks—allows you to have the base of the meal at the ready. Pull the rest of the meal together by following the tips below.

The 2-Week Turnaround dinner should contain around 400 calories, broken down as 1 grain/starchy veggie, 1 protein, 2 veggies, and 1 fat. Using the simple guidelines in the following 10 recipes (each ready in under 30 minutes sans some marinating time) will help you get supper together in a jiffy.

BUY PREPARED VEGGIES. Frozen vegetables are perfect for rush-hour meals. Be sure to purchase those that aren't cooked in sauce, so you can keep calories, fat, and sodium at bay. Try a variety of blends, and quickly steam or microwave for a side dish in minutes. Look for peeled and chopped vegetables in the produce section, or pick up some precut items at the salad bar. And don't forget pre-packed salads, which help to get supper on the table fast.

DOUBLE YOUR GRAINS. Having some parts of the meal cooked ahead saves time on rushed nights. Whenever you prepare long-cooking grains such as brown rice, wild rice, quinoa, or bulgur, be sure to double the amount needed. Stored in airtight containers, grains can be refrigerated for 3 to 5 days or frozen for up to 6 months.[1] Thaw frozen grains in the refrigerator and reheat in the microwave with 1 to 2 tablespoons water.

GET SAUCY. The right sauce can turn an ordinary serving of protein into a special treat. Stay clear of seasoning mixes or sauces that are loaded with sodium. Instead, reach for a jar of salsa, hoisin sauce, chutney, mole sauce or pesto. A smear of these sauces on a chicken breast, fillet of fish, chunk of tofu, or pork tenderloin creates a delicious meal in minutes.

CITRUS CHICKEN

¼ cup orange juice

1 tablespoon lemon juice

1 tablespoon lime juice

½ teaspoon dried thyme

4 boneless, skinless chicken breasts
(4 ounces each)

1½ cups reduced-sodium
chicken broth

1 cup quinoa, rinsed

2 red peppers, halved

2 large onions, each cut into
4 thick slices

1. Combine the orange juice, lemon juice, lime juice, and thyme in a large resealable bag. Add the chicken breasts, seal the bag, and refrigerate for 15 minutes to 8 hours.

2. Bring the chicken broth to a boil in a small saucepan over medium-high heat. Stir in the quinoa and reduce the heat to low. Cover and simmer for 20 minutes or until all the liquid is absorbed.

3. Preheat the grill or broiler. Remove the chicken from the marinade and grill or broil, turning once, for 15 minutes or until a thermometer inserted in the thickest portion registers 160°F and the juices run clear. During the last 7 minutes, grill or broil the peppers and onions until browned and tender.

4. Divide the chicken breast, peppers, onions, and quinoa among 4 plates.

MAKES 4 SERVINGS

PER SERVING: 345 calories; 4 g total fat; 1 g saturated fat; 41 g carbohydrate; 6 g fiber; 35 g protein; 66 mg cholesterol; 289 mg sodium

nutrition notes

◗ SKINLESS, BONELESS CHICKEN BREASTS *are a must-have in any healthy kitchen. This lean, protein-packed food is the go-to source for a quick and delicious meal.*

nutrition notes

NATIVE to the Mediterranean region, artichokes are loaded with fiber. In fact, a medium artichoke has more fiber than a cup of prunes!

CHICKEN AND ARTICHOKES

1 pound chicken breast tenders

1 package (9 ounces) frozen artichoke hearts, thawed

½ cup bottled low-fat Italian salad dressing

8 ounces whole grain penne pasta, cooked

4 cups baby arugula

1. Preheat the oven to 350°F. Coat a 13" × 9" baking dish with cooking spray.

2. Place the chicken and artichoke hearts in the dish and drizzle with the dressing.

3. Bake for 12 minutes or until a thermometer inserted in the thickest portion of the chicken registers 160°F and the juices run clear.

4. Place the pasta and arugula in a large bowl. Pour the chicken, artichokes, and dressing over the pasta. Toss to coat well.

MAKES 4 SERVINGS

PER SERVING: 415 calories; 8 g total fat; 1 g saturated fat; 47 g carbohydrate; 9 g fiber; 39 g protein; 66 mg cholesterol; 374 mg sodium

---

DIET DILEMMA: NEGATIVE SELF-TALK

Problem: It's that small voice inside your head—the one that says, "You will never lose weight," "Look in the mirror, you're so fat," and "Working out won't help—eat that cookie instead." This tiny voice can do huge damage to your diet and your self-esteem.

Solution: Think about what that voice is telling you—would you ever say those things to your best friend? Absolutely not, so why would you say them to yourself? When you start thinking negative thoughts, do something for yourself—take a walk, read a book, call a friend—and ignore the voice. Also try sending yourself positive internal messages. Be your own best cheerleader, instead, and you'll find that your motivation and your weight loss will increase.

VEGETABLE PASTA

1 can (14.5 ounces) basil, garlic, and oregano-flavored diced tomatoes

1 package (9 ounces) frozen quartered artichoke hearts, thawed

¼ cup pitted kalamata olives, finely chopped

1 tablespoon no-salt-added tomato paste

8 ounces whole grain mini rigatoni pasta, cooked

¼ cup chopped fresh basil

12 ounces leftover or deli roast beef

1. Combine the tomatoes, artichokes, olives, and tomato paste in a medium saucepan. Bring to a simmer over medium heat and cook for 5 minutes or until flavored through and artichokes are tender.

2. Toss with the pasta and basil in a large bowl until combined. Serve with the roast beef.

MAKES 4 SERVINGS

PER SERVING: 394 calories; 8 g total fat; 2 g saturated fat; 49 g carbohydrate; 9 g fiber; 31 g protein; 45 mg cholesterol; 789 mg sodium

NOTE: This recipe is a little high in sodium (you want to aim for no more than 600 to 650 milligrams per meal), so be sure to work this recipe into your daily total of 2,300 milligrams of sodium by selecting recipes for the remaining meals that are around 300 to 400 milligrams each.

nutrition notes

● OLIVES *are concentrated sources of healthy monounsaturated fats. And since they pack such a flavor punch, you can use them sparingly to save calories.*

nutrition notes

● ONCE PER OUNCE, *pork tenderloin has less fat than chicken breast!*

HOISIN PORK

1 pork tenderloin (about 12 ounces)

2 tablespoons hoisin sauce

3 heads baby bok choy, halved lengthwise

4 carrots, halved lengthwise

4 cups cooked brown rice

1. Preheat the oven to 450°F.

2. Place the pork in a roasting pan. Brush with the hoisin sauce. Roast for 15 minutes. Scatter the bok choy and carrots around the pork. Roast for 5 to 10 minutes longer or until a thermometer inserted in the center of the pork registers 155°F. Let stand for 5 minutes before slicing.

3. Divide the pork and vegetables among 4 plates and serve each with 1 cup cooked brown rice.

MAKES 4 SERVINGS

PER SERVING: 359 calories; 4 g total fat; 1 g saturated fat; 55 g carbohydrate; 6 g fiber; 25 g protein; 56 mg cholesterol; 263 mg sodium

● LOADED WITH FIBER, *protein, and nutrients, beans are darn near perfect. One cup has 12 grams of filling fiber—about half of the recommended daily amount.*

PORK CUTLETS MOLE

1 tablespoon olive oil

2 medium zucchini, diced

2 teaspoons chili powder

1 cup frozen corn

1 cup canned unsalted black beans, drained

4 boneless pork loin cutlets (1 pound)

1 cup prepared mole sauce

1. Heat the oil in a large saucepan over medium heat. Add the zucchini and cook 4 minutes. Stir in the chili powder and cook 1 minute. Stir in the corn and black beans, cover, and cook for 6 minutes or until the vegetables are tender.

2. Meanwhile, heat a nonstick skillet coated with cooking spray over medium heat. Cook the pork for 3 minutes. Turn the pork, add the sauce, and cook for 4 to 5 minutes more or until the pork is no longer pink. Serve with the vegetables.

MAKES 4 SERVINGS

PER SERVING: 379 calories; 15 g total fat; 2 g saturated fat; 29 g carbohydrate; 8 g fiber; 34 g protein; 75 mg cholesterol; 158 mg sodium

SHRIMP PASTA PRIMAVERA

8 ounces whole grain penne pasta

1 pound frozen raw medium shrimp, thawed

1 bag (16 ounces) frozen broccoli, onions, mushrooms, and peppers

½ cup fat-free plain Greek-style yogurt

¼ cup low-fat Caesar salad dressing

2 tablespoons shredded Parmesan cheese

1. Prepare the pasta according to package directions, adding the shrimp and vegetables during the last 3 minutes of cooking. Drain well.

2. Meanwhile, whisk together the yogurt and salad dressing in a large bowl. Add the hot pasta and vegetables and toss to coat well. Sprinkle with the cheese.

MAKES 4 SERVINGS

PER SERVING: 405 calories; 4 g total fat; 1 g saturated fat; 49 g carbohydrate; 5 g fiber; 38 g protein; 175 mg cholesterol; 423 mg sodium

nutrition notes

● LOOK FOR LOW-FAT *Caesar dressings with no more than 150 calories, 2 g of saturated fat, and 200 mg of sodium per 2 tablespoons.*

CHAPTER 6 ○ DINNERS

● CANNELLINI BEANS *are considered the Italian kidney bean. They're not only an excellent source of folate, they're also a good source of iron and fiber.*

CRISPY BAKED SCALLOPS

¾ cup whole wheat panko bread crumbs, finely crushed

2 teaspoons lemon zest

4 teaspoons olive oil

1¼ pounds sea scallops

1 pound steamed broccoli florets

1½ cups canned unsalted cannellini beans, drained

⅓ cup reduced-fat balsamic vinaigrette

1. Preheat the oven to 450°F. Coat a baking sheet with cooking spray.

2. Toss together the bread crumbs and lemon zest in a large bowl. Gradually add the oil, stirring until evenly coated. One at a time, toss the scallops in the crumbs and place on the baking sheet. Mound any remaining crumbs on top of the scallops.

3. Bake for 4 to 8 minutes (depending on the size) or until opaque. Toss the broccoli, cannellini beans, and vinaigrette in a bowl. Serve with the scallops.

MAKES 4 SERVINGS

PER SERVING: 338 calories; 8 g total fat; 1 g saturated fat; 37 g carbohydrate; 9 g fiber; 34 g protein; 47 mg cholesterol; 548 mg sodium

nutrition notes

● QUICK-COOKING, *rich, and nutty whole wheat couscous offers more fiber, nutrients, and flavor than white couscous.*

● SESAME OIL *is high in vitamin E, which can help lower cholesterol. And because it has such a strong flavor, a little goes a long way.*

PESTO FISH

1 cod fillet (about 6 ounces)

1 tablespoon reduced-fat refrigerated pesto

½ cup low-sodium chicken broth

⅓ cup whole wheat couscous

⅛ teaspoon salt

4 ounces green beans, trimmed and steamed

1. Preheat the oven to 400°F. Coat a baking sheet with cooking spray.

2. Place the cod on a baking sheet and brush with the pesto. Roast for 6 to 8 minutes or until fish flakes easily.

3. Meanwhile, bring the broth, couscous, and salt to a boil over high heat. Remove from the heat and let stand 5 minutes.

4. Serve the cod with the couscous and steamed green beans.

MAKES 1 SERVING

PER SERVING: 373 calories; 7 g total fat; 1 g saturated fat; 40 g carbohydrate; 9 g fiber; 39 g protein; 77 mg cholesterol; 606 mg sodium

ASIAN FISH PACKETS

4 tilapia fillets (1¼ pounds)

1 cup peapods, cut lengthwise into strips

1 cup red bell pepper strips

1 cup shredded carrots

4 tablespoons Asian stir-fry sauce

4 teaspoons toasted sesame oil

2 cups hot cooked brown rice

1. Preheat the oven to 425°F. Set out four 16" lengths of aluminum foil or parchment paper.

2. Place a fillet in the center of each. Top with the peapods, peppers, and carrots. Drizzle with the stir-fry sauce and sesame oil. Fold the foil into packets, making a tight seal; place on a baking sheet.

3. Bake for 22 minutes, or until the fish flakes easily, opening carefully to avoid the escaping steam. Serve with the rice.

MAKES 4 SERVINGS

PER SERVING: 333 calories; 8 g total fat; 2 g saturated fat; 33 g carbohydrate; 4 g fiber; 33 g protein; 71 mg cholesterol; 490 mg sodium

MOROCCAN KEBABS

½ cup sun-dried tomato
salad dressing

½ teaspoon mild smoked paprika

1 package (12 ounces drained weight)
extra-firm low-fat tofu, cut into
1½" cubes

2 red bell peppers, cut into 1" pieces

2 medium zucchini, cut into 1" pieces

1 medium red onion, cut into 1" pieces

10 kalamata olives, chopped

2 cups cooked quinoa

1. Stir together the salad dressing and paprika in a large shallow bowl. Add the tofu and marinate for 20 minutes. Alternately thread the peppers, zucchini, red onion, and tofu on eight 10" skewers, reserving any dressing. Preheat a grill or grill pan to medium-high heat.

2. Grill the skewers for 10 to 12 minutes or until the vegetables and tofu are browned, basting occasionally with the dressing.

3. Stir the olives into the quinoa. Serve with the skewers and reserved dressing.

MAKES 4 SERVINGS

PER SERVING: 316 calories; 13 g total fat; 1 g saturated fat; 37 g carbohydrate; 6 g fiber; 15 g protein; 0 mg cholesterol; 542 mg sodium

nutrition notes

● TOFU *(aka bean curd) is a nutritious and protein-packed meat alternative made from the curds of soybean milk. Look for tofu listing calcium sulfate on the ingredients panel.*

SNACKS AND
DESSERTS

CHAPTER 7 ∘ SNACKS AND DESSERTS

"THERE ARE FEW THINGS THAT YOU CAN'T DO AS LONG AS YOU ARE WILLING TO APPLY YOURSELF."

—GREG LEMOND

CHILLED CUCUMBER SOUP

2 large cucumbers (12 ounces each), peeled and seeded

⅛ teaspoon salt

1 large apple, peeled, cored, and coarsely chopped

1 cup low-fat buttermilk

½ cup ice cubes

¼ cup reduced-fat sour cream

2 to 3 teaspoons chopped fresh mint

1 teaspoon honey

Pinch of ground white pepper

1 cup crumbled reduced-fat feta cheese

2 tablespoons pine nuts, toasted

SERVE THIS SOUP as a snack or as the perfect light summer lunch with a crisp green salad and grilled chicken. If you like, substitute a juicy ripe pear for the apple or fresh dill for the mint. If you plan to make this ahead, blend in the mint at the last minute because the flavor will intensify as it stands. *This recipe makes a good pre/postworkout snack.*

TOTAL TIME: 15 MINUTES

1. Cut 1 of the cucumbers into ¼" cubes. Place in a small bowl and toss with the salt. Set aside for 15 minutes.

2. Cut the remaining cucumber into 1" chunks and place in a blender. Add the apple, buttermilk, ice cubes, sour cream, mint, honey, and pepper. Blend for 1 to 2 minutes, or until smooth.

3. Divide among 4 bowls. Top each with one-quarter of the reserved cucumber, ¼ cup of the cheese, and ½ tablespoon of the pine nuts.

MAKES 4 SERVINGS

PER SERVING: 191 calories; 8 g total fat; 4 g saturated fat; 20 g carbohydrate; 5 g fiber; 12 g protein; 17 mg cholesterol; 651 mg sodium

WHITE BEAN DIP

"IF YOU LIKE hummus, you will love this white bean dip. It's great for parties and perfect for dipping veggies! This is always in my fridge! *This recipe makes a good pre/post workout snack.*"

TOTAL TIME: 10 MINUTES

1. Combine the beans, parsley, cheese, lemon juice, garlic, oil, and 1 tablespoon of water in a food processor or blender. Process until smooth.

2. Serve with the pita chips. Store any remaining dip in an airtight container in the refrigerator.

MAKES 6 SERVINGS

PER SERVING: 214 calories; 8 g fat; 0 g saturated fat; 30 g carbohydrate; 3 g fiber; 7 g protein; 3 mg cholesterol; 109 mg sodium

1 can (19 ounces) cannellini beans, rinsed and drained

¼ cup parsley

¼ cup grated Parmesan cheese

2 tablespoons lemon juice

2 cloves garlic

1 tablespoon olive oil

6 ounces low-fat baked pita chips

CHAPTER 7 ∘ SNACKS AND DESSERTS

WATERMELON FETA STACKS

1 medium cucumber, cut into 24 slices

8 ounces seedless, rindless watermelon

3 ounces crumbled feta or goat cheese

1½ tablespoons fresh lime juice

1 tablespoon honey

2 teaspoons finely chopped fresh mint

SWEET, SALTY, AND creamy—these stacks cover all the bases. Assemble and refrigerate the stacks up to 3 hours in advance. Then drizzle with the honey lime sauce just before serving. Scatter the platter with fresh mint leaves for a festive occasion. *This recipe makes a good pre/postworkout snack.*

TOTAL TIME: 15 MINUTES

1. Arrange 12 cucumber slices on a serving plate. Cut the watermelon into four 1½" cubes. Cut each cube into 6 slices.

2. Place 1 watermelon slice on each cucumber round. Scatter half of the cheese on top. Place the remaining cucumbers slices on top, pressing down gently to level the cheese. Top each with a watermelon slice. Scatter the remaining cheese on top.

3. Whisk together the lime juice, honey, and mint in a small bowl until blended. Right before serving, drizzle the honey mixture over the stacks.

MAKES 3 SERVINGS

PER SERVING: 182 calories; 10 g total fat; 6 g saturated fat; 16 g carbohydrate; 2 g fiber; 10 g protein; 28 mg cholesterol; 307 mg sodium

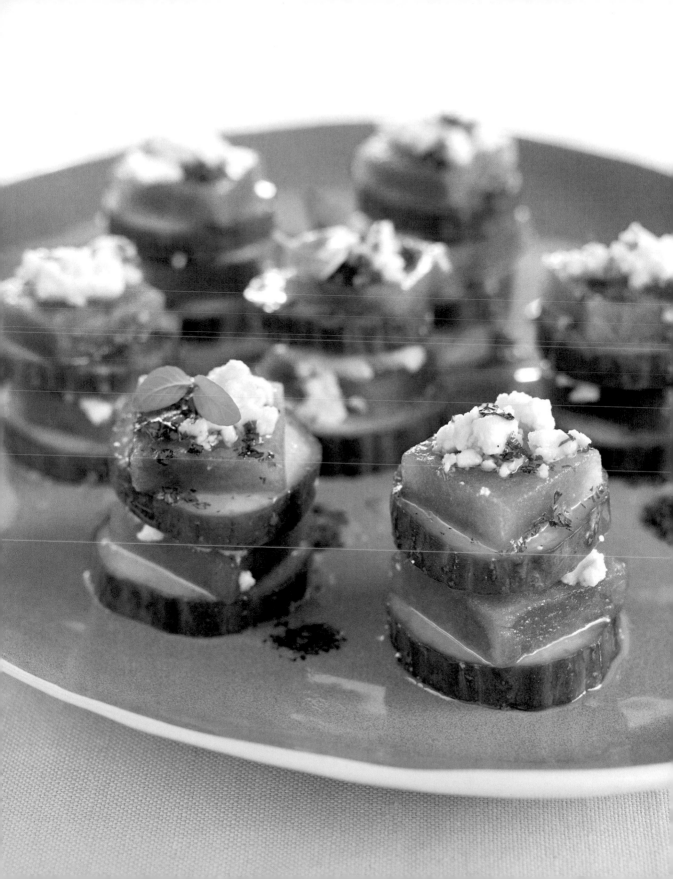

GOAT CHEESE WITH BERRY COMPOTE

2 ounces chilled fresh goat cheese

1 tablespoon honey

1 teaspoon fresh lemon juice

½ teaspoon grated fresh ginger

⅛ teaspoon ground allspice

1 cup fresh blueberries

1 cup fresh raspberries

1 teaspoon fresh mint, cut into thin slivers

CREAMY MILD GOAT cheese is the perfect accompaniment for fruit. Get creative and vary the fruit according to the season. Fresh plums, peaches, strawberries, cherries, oranges, figs, and ripe pears are all winning possibilities. *This recipe makes a good pre/postworkout snack.*

TOTAL TIME: 15 MINUTES

1. Slice the cheese while it is cold into 4 rounds (about ⅜" thick) and divide between 2 plates. Let stand for 15 minutes to soften.

2. Meanwhile, stir together the honey, lemon juice, ginger, and allspice in a medium bowl until blended. Gently toss in the blueberries, raspberries, and mint. Spoon onto the cheese and serve.

PER SERVING: 211 calories; 9 g total fat; 6 g saturated fat; 28 g carbohydrate; 6 g fiber; 8 g protein; 22 mg cholesterol; 148 mg sodium

METABOLISM BOOSTER: KICK UP CALCIUM

Calcium not only strengthens your teeth and bones, it may also help shrink your waistline. While studies haven't yet proven that eating calcium-rich dairy foods speeds up metabolism, these foods can definitely help you lose weight in other ways. In one study, people who followed reduced-calorie diets and increased their dairy intake to three servings per day lost more weight than people who didn't consume enough calcium.[1] It's still not clear why this mineral helps with weight loss, but one theory is that it may boost metabolism, which can prompt our bodies to burn fat.[2] So go ahead and start including that low-fat yogurt and fat-free milk with your meals, if you aren't already taking advantage of calcium's myriad health benefits.

HONEYED YOGURT DIP
WITH ORANGE SECTIONS

G REEK-STYLE YOGURT WILL result in a thicker dip, but if it's not available, regular fat-free yogurt will work well also. If you have the time, place the regular yogurt in a coffee filter in a sieve over a bowl and chill for 1 to 3 hours. This will release some of the liquid, making a thicker yogurt that's more like the Greek-style. *This recipe makes a good pre/postworkout snack.*

TOTAL TIME: 5 MINUTES

1. Mix together the yogurt, honey, and orange zest in a small bowl.

2. Serve with orange sections to dip into the yogurt.

MAKES 1 SERVING

PER SERVING: 237 calories; 0 g total fat; 0 g saturated fat; 39 g carbohydrate; 4 g fiber; 21 g protein; 0 mg cholesterol; 85 mg sodium

8 ounces fat-free plain Greek-style yogurt

2 teaspoons honey

1 tablespoon orange zest

1 small orange, peeled and separated into sections

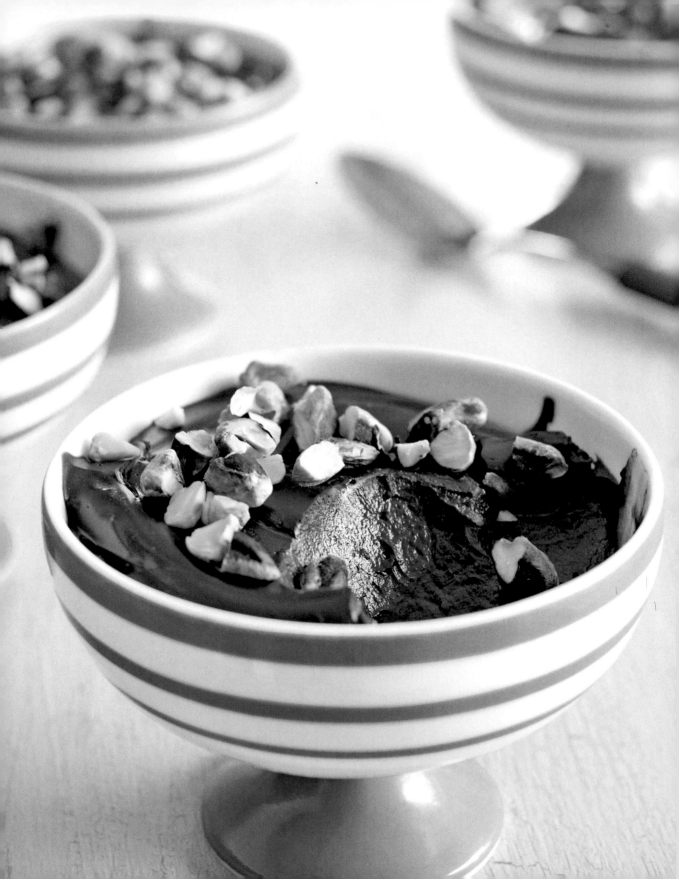

CHOCOLATE PUDDING

THIS RECIPE TAKES some stirring, but the result will be worth it! Any nut will work, so try almonds, pecans, or walnuts. Store extra pudding in the refrigerator for up to 3 days.

TOTAL TIME: 10 MINUTES PLUS CHILLING TIME

1. Place the cornstarch, cocoa powder, and sugar in a medium saucepan. Whisk in 1 cup of the milk until smooth.

2. Cook over medium heat, stirring constantly, while gradually adding the remaining 1½ cups milk. Continue stirring until the mixture comes to a boil. Boil for 1 minute, stirring constantly.

3. Remove from the heat and pour into 4 cups. Sprinkle with the pistachios. Chill for 20 minutes, or until ready to serve.

MAKES 4 SERVINGS

PER SERVING: 166 calories; 4 g total fat; 1 g saturated fat; 29 g carbohydrate; 2 g fiber; 8 g protein; 3 mg cholesterol; 67 mg sodium

¼ cup cornstarch

¼ cup unsweetened cocoa powder

3 tablespoons sugar

2½ cups fat-free milk, divided

3 tablespoons unsalted shelled pistachio nuts, chopped

MANGO SORBET

1 cup frozen diced mango

1 cup fat-free half-and-half

1 cup low-fat plain yogurt, divided

¼ cup orange juice

4 (0.35 ounce) packets powdered stevia or 4 packets Splenda

½ teaspoon vanilla extract

STOCK UP ON frozen mangoes, and keep this satisfying dessert on hand for those sweet cravings. Substitute frozen peaches, strawberries, raspberries, or cherries for the mango and you'll never be bored with dessert. Spoon the frozen mixture into ice-pop molds for a treat on the fly. You can double this recipe to serve 4.

TOTAL TIME: 15 MINUTES PLUS CHILLING TIME

Process the mango in a food processor until finely chopped, pulsing and scraping down the sides of the bowl. Add the half-and-half, yogurt, orange juice, stevia or Splenda, and vanilla extract and process until smooth. Freeze in an ice-cream maker according to the manufacturer's instructions.

MAKES 2 SERVINGS

PER SERVING: 215 calories; 0 g total fat; 0 g saturated fat; 43 g carbohydrate; 2 g fiber; 10 g protein; 3 mg cholesterol; 168 mg sodium

NOTE. Food processor freezing: If you don't have an ice-cream maker, pour the mixture into a 9″ × 9″ metal pan, cover, and freeze for about 3 hours, or until just frozen. Scrape into a food processor and process until smooth and fluffy. Return to the pan and freeze for 1 to 2 hours, or until firm.

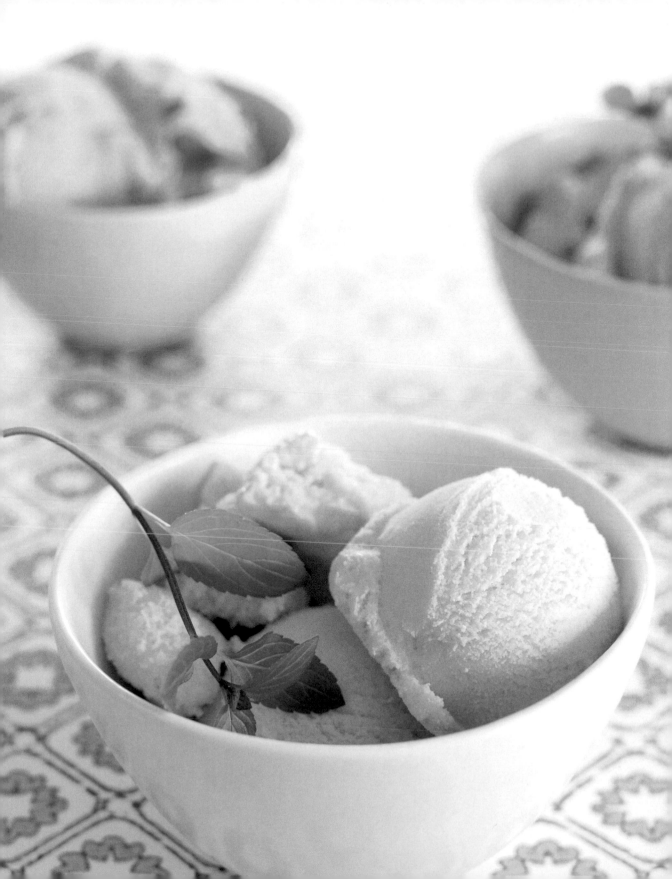

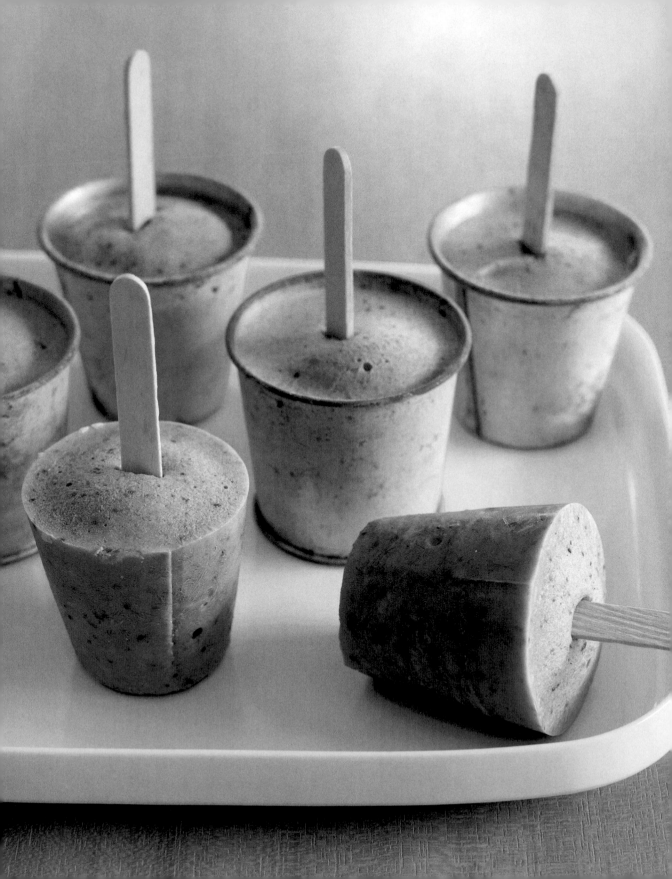

FROZEN BANANA YOGURT POP

I F POSSIBLE, USE ripe bananas, which will result in sweeter pops. Change up these pops by substituting raspberries, blueberries, or peaches for the strawberries. *This recipe makes a good pre/postworkout snack.*

TOTAL TIME: 3 MINUTES PLUS FREEZING TIME

1. Combine the yogurt, strawberries, banana, vanilla extract, and nectar or honey in a blender. Process until smooth.

2. Pour the mixture into 4 ice-pop molds or paper cups. Place an ice-pop stick in the middle of each cup and freeze for 2 hours, or until solid.

3. To serve, remove from the molds or peel away the paper cup.

MAKES 4 SERVINGS

PER SERVING: 178 calories; 0 g total fat; 0 g saturated fat; 29 g carbohydrate; 2 g fiber; 15 g protein; 0 mg cholesterol; 64 mg sodium

3 cups fat-free plain Greek-style yogurt

2 cups frozen unsweetened strawberries

1 medium banana

2 teaspoons vanilla extract

2 tablespoons agave nectar or honey

VANILLA AND ORANGE YOGURT CUP

¾ cup fat-free plain yogurt

1 tablespoon fresh orange juice

1 teaspoon vanilla extract

2 teaspoons agave nectar or honey

1 teaspoon orange zest

½ cup fresh raspberries

2 tablespoons low-fat granola

O RANGE, LEMON, AND lime zest—the thin, brightly colored portion of a citrus peel—add great flavor to dishes. There are several tools that make zesting easy, the most popular being a microplane rasp or grater (the smallest side of your box grater). *This recipe makes a good pre/postworkout snack.*

TOTAL TIME: 5 MINUTES

1. Combine the yogurt, orange juice, vanilla extract, nectar or honey, and orange zest in a medium bowl.

2. Place the raspberries (set aside a few for garnish) in a large parfait glass or serving bowl. Sprinkle with 1 tablespoon of the granola. Top with the yogurt mixture and the remaining 1 tablespoon granola. Garnish with the reserved raspberries.

MAKES 1 SERVING

PER SERVING: 215 calories; 1 g total fat; 0 g saturated fat; 45 g carbohydrate; 5 g fiber; 9 g protein; 4 mg cholesterol; 132 mg sodium

LEMON BUTTERMILK PANNA COTTAS

THESE COOL, CREAMY desserts seem to melt in your mouth. A great make-ahead dessert, these are perfect for the summer, as they're practically no-cook. Light, refreshing, quick, easy, and low in calories—what's not to love?

TOTAL TIME: 15 MINUTES PLUS CHILLING TIME

1. Sprinkle the gelatin over ¼ cup water. Let stand for 2 minutes to allow the gelatin to absorb the water and soften.

2. Heat ½ cup of the half-and-half for 3 minutes in a large saucepan over medium heat. Reduce the heat to low and whisk in the gelatin. Cook, stirring, for 1 minute, or until the gelatin dissolves. Remove the saucepan from the heat and stir in the buttermilk, nectar or honey, lemon zest, and remaining ¼ cup half-and-half.

3. Pour the buttermilk mixture into six 4-ounce ramekins or 6-ounce custard cups. Place the ramekins in a large baking dish and cover the dish with plastic wrap. Refrigerate for at least 4 hours or overnight, or until well chilled and set.

4. Place the spreadable fruit in a small microwaveable bowl. Microwave on high for 30 seconds and stir until smooth, then stir in 2 teaspoons water. Gently stir in the raspberries.

5. To unmold the panna cottas, run the tip of a knife around the edge of each ramekin. With your hand, sharply tap the side of each ramekin to break the seal. Invert onto 6 dessert plates and top with the raspberries.

MAKES 6 SERVINGS

PER SERVING: 183 calories; 1 g total fat; 1 g saturated fat; 40 g carbohydrate; 3 g fiber; 5 g protein; 5 mg cholesterol; 132 mg sodium

1 envelope unflavored gelatin

¾ cup fat-free half-and-half, divided

2 cups low-fat buttermilk

½ cup agave nectar or honey

2 teaspoons lemon zest

¼ cup seedless raspberry spreadable fruit

1 pint fresh raspberries

MINI LEMON CAKE WITH BERRIES

¼ teaspoon apple cider vinegar

3¼ cups fat-free milk, divided

5 tablespoons unbleached all-purpose flour

3 tablespoons sugar

1½ teaspoons cornstarch

¼ teaspoon baking powder

⅛ teaspoon baking soda

Pinch of salt

1 tablespoon + 1 teaspoon canola oil

1 teaspoon lemon juice

1 teaspoon lemon zest

1 cup fresh raspberries, strawberries, or blueberries

USE YOUR FAVORITE berry or a mix of several berries to serve with these light yet extremely flavorful cakes. Try black and red raspberries or all blackberries.

TOTAL TIME: 30 MINUTES

1. Preheat the oven to 350°F. Coat 4 cupcake or muffin cups with cooking spray.

2. Combine the vinegar and ¼ cup of the milk in a large bowl and mix thoroughly. Add the flour, sugar, cornstarch, baking powder, baking soda, salt, oil, lemon juice, and lemon zest. Stir until just blended.

3. Divide the batter among the cups. Bake for 18 minutes, or until springy to the touch.

4. Place 1 cake on each of 4 plates. Surround each cake with ¼ cup of the berries and serve with ¾ cup milk.

MAKES 4 SERVINGS

PER SERVING: 203 calories; 5 g total fat; 0 g saturated fat; 32 g carbohydrate; 2 g fiber; 9 g protein; 3 mg cholesterol; 214 mg sodium

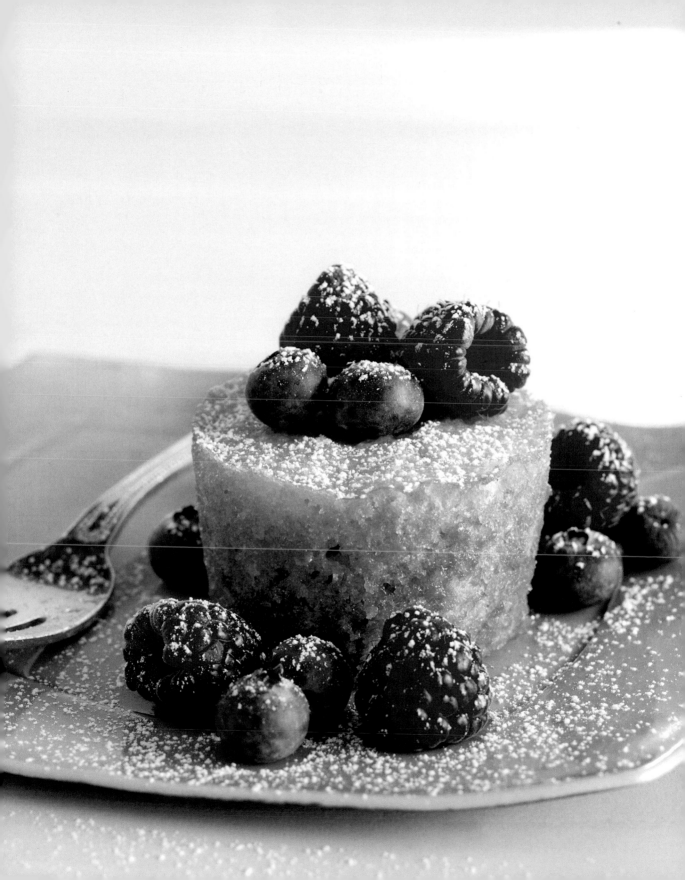

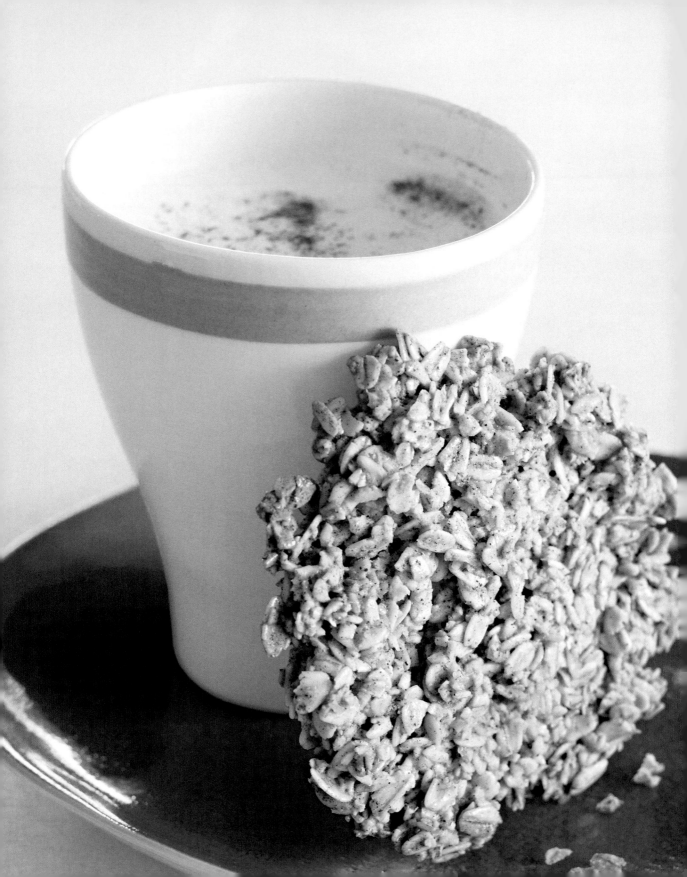

OATMEAL COOKIE WITH WARM MILK

MAKING JUST 4 cookies ensures that there are no leftovers. If you desire, bake one cookie at a time, storing the batter in the refrigerator for at least a week.

TOTAL TIME: 15 MINUTES

1. Preheat the oven to 350°F. Coat a baking sheet with cooking spray.

2. Combine the oats, 1 tablespoon milk, oil, baking powder, honey, cinnamon, and salt in a food processor. Pulse on and off 6 times, or until well blended and the oats are in small pieces.

3. Divide the dough into 4 equal pieces. Place on the baking sheet and flatten with the palm of your hand.

4. Bake for 12 minutes, or until golden brown on the edges. Serve each cookie with 1 cup of warm milk sprinkled with cinnamon, if desired.

MAKES 4 SERVINGS

PER SERVING: 207 calories; 5 g total fat; 1 g saturated fat; 31 g carbohydrate; 2 g fiber; 11 g protein; 5 mg cholesterol; 166 mg sodium

¾ cup old-fashioned rolled oats

1 tablespoon fat-free milk

1 tablespoon olive oil

½ teaspoon baking powder

2 tablespoons honey

¼ teaspoon ground cinnamon

Pinch of salt

4 cups fat-free milk, warmed

APPLE SLICES WITH SPICED RICOTTA DIP

½ cup fat-free ricotta cheese

½ tablespoon smooth peanut butter

Pinch of cinnamon

1 small apple, cored and sliced

I F YOU ARE a fan of chunky peanut butter, substitute it for the smooth for a little added crunch in this tasty dip. *This recipe makes a good pre/postworkout snack.*

TOTAL TIME: 5 MINUTES

1. Stir together the ricotta, peanut butter, and cinnamon in a small bowl until smooth.

2. Serve with the apple slices to dip into the peanut butter mixture.

MAKES 1 SERVING

PER SERVING: 225 calories; 4 g total fat; 1 g saturated fat; 32 g carbohydrate; 4 g fiber; 12 g protein; 20 mg cholesterol; 168 mg sodium

PEANUT BUTTER AND CHOCOLATE ENERGY BARS

"I CREATED THIS ENERGY bar because I was tired of the expensive protein and energy bars full of chemicals and additives. I couldn't find many that were all natural, tasty, and affordable. This recipe satisfies my sweet tooth and is a quick pick-me-up anytime of day. My kids and their friends always ask for them."

TOTAL TIME: 15 MINUTES

1. Line a 13″ × 9″ baking pan with wax paper. Combine the cereal, oats, almonds, sunflower seeds, walnuts, chocolate chips, and flaxseed in a large bowl. Set aside.

2. Combine the nectar or honey, brown sugar, peanut butter, butter, and salt in a small saucepan. Bring to a low boil and cook for 3 minutes. Remove from the heat and stir in the vanilla extract.

3. Pour quickly over the cereal mixture, stirring to coat well. (The chocolate chips will melt.)

4. With wet fingers, press the mixture into the pan. Let cool for 5 minutes. Cut into 24 rectangles. Store at room temperature in an airtight container for up to 5 days. Freeze for up to 2 months.

MAKES 24 SERVINGS

PER SERVING: 205 calories; 11 g total fat; 2 g saturated fat; 25 g carbohydrate; 2 g fiber; 4 g protein; 3 mg cholesterol; 54 mg sodium

2½ cups puffed wheat cereal

1½ cups old-fashioned rolled oats

½ cup slivered almonds, lightly chopped

½ cup sunflower seeds

½ cup chopped walnuts

½ cup 60% cocoa chocolate chips

¼ cup ground flaxseed

¾ cup agave nectar or honey

¾ cup brown sugar

½ cup natural peanut butter

2 tablespoons butter

¼ teaspoon salt

1 teaspoon vanilla extract

SKILLET FRUIT CRISP

2 tablespoons cornstarch or arrowroot

1 teaspoon butter

3 medium plums or peaches, pitted and cut into thin wedges

2 tablespoons lemon juice

2 tablespoons honey

Pinch of ground cardamom

½ cup low-fat granola

3 cups fat-free Greek-style yogurt

HERE'S A DELICIOUS way to serve fresh fruit—spiked with cardamom and topped with a crunchy topping and creamy yogurt. For ease, sprinkle the granola over the cooked fruit mixture and serve directly from the skillet. For a special presentation, divide the fruit mixture among 4 bowls, top with the yogurt, and sprinkle with the granola. *The recipe makes a good pre/postworkout snack.*

TOTAL TIME: 15 MINUTES

1. Whisk together the cornstarch or arrowroot and 1 tablespoon water in a small bowl until well blended. Set aside.

2. Heat the butter in a medium skillet over medium-high heat. Add the plums or peaches and cook, stirring gently, for 3 minutes, or until lightly browned.

3. Drizzle with the lemon juice, honey, and cardamom and cook for 1 minute. Whisk the cornstarch mixture until smooth and stir into the skillet, stirring gently but constantly until thickened. Remove from the heat and sprinkle with the granola.

4. Divide into 4 bowls and top each with ¾ cup of the yogurt.

MAKES 4 SERVINGS

PER SERVING: 216 calories; 2 g total fat; 1 g saturated fat; 35 g carbohydrate; 2 g fiber; 16 g protein; 3 mg cholesterol; 93 mg sodium

BAKED APPLE WITH YOGURT SAUCE

ALTHOUGH THIS RECIPE works with any type of apple, try it with a crisp variety, such as Honeycrisp, Granny Smith, or Gala, which will yield an ideal consistency after baking.

TOTAL TIME: 35 MINUTES

1. Heat the oven to 375°F. Coat an 8″ x 8″ baking pan with cooking spray. Place the apple halves, skin sides down, in the pan. Drizzle with 1 teaspoon of the nectar and sprinkle with the ginger, nutmeg, and cloves. Bake for 30 minutes, or until tender.

2. Meanwhile, stir together the yogurt and the remaining 2 teaspoons nectar. Serve the cooked apple with the yogurt sauce.

MAKES 1 SERVING

PER SERVING: 245 calories; 0 g total fat; 0 g saturated fat; 48 g carbohydrate; 4 g fiber; 15 g protein; 0 mg cholesterol; 64 mg sodium

1 medium apple, halved and cored

1 tablespoon agave nectar, divided

Pinch of ground ginger

Pinch of ground nutmeg

Pinch of ground cloves

¾ cup fat-free plain Greek-style yogurt

BROILED PEACH
WITH VANILLA CUSTARD

1 small peach, cut in half
   and pit removed

1 tablespoon cornstarch

1 teaspoon honey

¼ teaspoon vanilla extract

1 cup fat-free milk

IF YOU LIKE a thicker sauce, prepare the custard and refrigerate it for at least 30 minutes before serving. Many fruits are delicious broiled; try pears or apricots.

TOTAL TIME: 10 MINUTES

1. Preheat the oven to broil. Coat an 8" x 8" baking pan with cooking spray. Place the peach halves, cut sides down, in the pan. Spray the peach with cooking spray. Broil for 5 minutes, or until the skin is lightly browned.

2. Meanwhile, combine the cornstarch, honey, and vanilla extract in a medium saucepan. Whisk in the milk until there are no lumps. Cook over medium heat, stirring constantly, for 5 minutes, or until the mixture comes to a boil. Boil for 1 minute, stirring constantly.

3. Serve the peach smothered with the warm or chilled custard.

MAKES 1 SERVING

PER SERVING: 190 calories; 0 g total fat; 0 g saturated fat; 37 g carbohydrate; 2 g fiber; 10 g protein; 3 mg cholesterol; 131 mg sodium

CHOCOLATE AND PEANUT BUTTER SHAKE

S TEVIA IS AN herb native to South America that works wonderfully as a sweetener and is now available in many forms. Look for it in powder or liquid forms in the natural section of your market or in packet form with the other sweeteners. *This recipe makes a good pre/postworkout snack.*

TOTAL TIME: 5 MINUTES PLUS FREEZING TIME

Place ½ cup of the milk into ice cube trays and freeze for 1 hour, or until solid. Combine the milk cubes, peanut butter, cocoa powder, stevia, and the remaining ½ cup milk in a blender. Process until smooth.

MAKES 1 SERVING

PER SERVING: 202 calories; 8 g total fat; 2 g saturated fat; 21 g carbohydrate; 2 g fiber; 14 g protein; 3 mg cholesterol; 204 mg sodium

1 cup fat-free milk

1 tablespoon natural peanut butter

½ tablespoon unsweetened cocoa powder

3 packets stevia

DIET DILEMMA: MINDLESS MUNCHING

Problem: You're sitting in front of the TV, and the bag of chips you just opened is suddenly empty. Or you find yourself wandering past your coworker's candy dish multiple times per day. This is mindless munching—snacking that you do without even noticing. The bad news is that these small snacks can add up to major calories—and weight gain.

Solution: Set aside designated meal and snack times, and don't allow yourself to snack at any other time. (And don't eat in front of the TV or computer.) The good news: This plan is designed with three satisfying meals and two snacks, so you can lock yourself into eating delicious foods five times a day.

FROZEN CINNAMON LATTE

1 cup fat-free milk

1 small ripe pear, quartered and cored

1½ teaspoons agave nectar or honey

½ teaspoon cinnamon

Pinch of salt

REMEMBER TO FREEZE the milk in ice-cube trays ahead of time, so this snack can be made in a couple of minutes. *This recipe makes a good pre/postworkout snack.*

TOTAL TIME: 2 MINUTES PLUS FREEZING TIME

1. Place ½ cup of the milk into ice-cube trays and freeze for 1 hour, or until solid.

2. Combine the milk cubes, pear, nectar or honey, cinnamon, salt, and the remaining ½ cup milk in a blender. Process until smooth.

MAKES 1 SERVING

PER SERVING: 202 calories; 0 g total fat; 0 g saturated fat; 44 g carbohydrate; 5 g fiber; 9 g protein; 5 mg cholesterol; 104 mg sodium

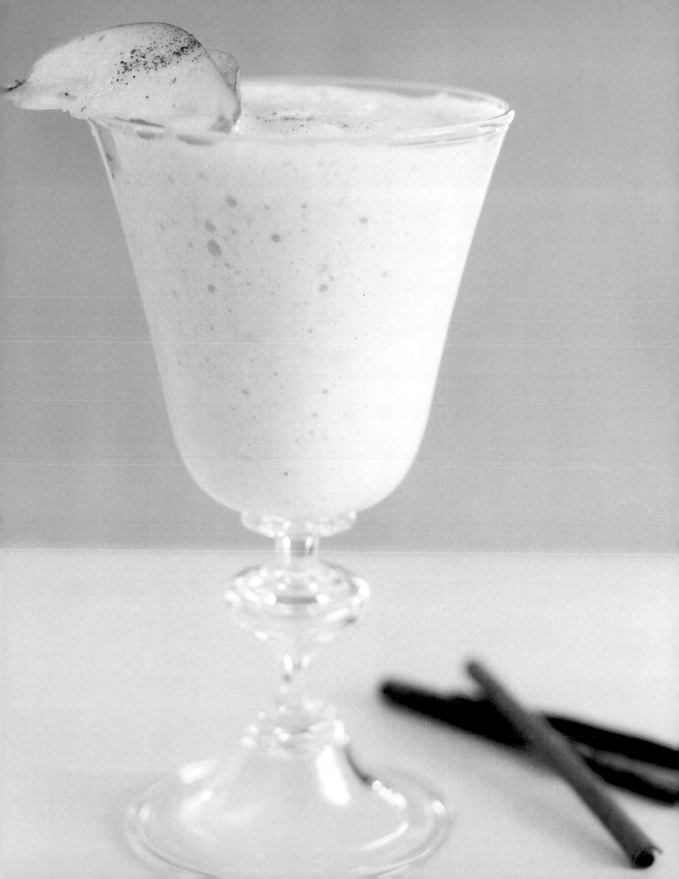

MEXICAN CHOCOLATE MILK

1 cup light soy milk or unsweetened almond milk

2 teaspoons unsweetened cocoa powder

1 teaspoon agave nectar or honey

½ teaspoon cinnamon, divided

1 pear

COCOA POWDER IS a great way to get the antioxidants present in chocolate without all the fat. Here, chocolate and cinnamon combine for a classic Mexican drink.

TOTAL TIME: 5 MINUTES

1. Whisk together the soy milk, cocoa powder, nectar or honey, and ¼ teaspoon of the cinnamon in a small saucepan. Cook over medium heat for 4 minutes or until hot.

2. Pour into a mug and sprinkle with the remaining ¼ teaspoon cinnamon. Serve with the pear.

MAKES 1 SERVING

PER SERVING: 177 calories; 3 g total fat; 1 g saturated fat; 38 g carbohydrate; 6 g fiber; 5 g protein; 0 mg cholesterol; 112 mg sodium

CREAMY ICED COFFEE

"I LOVE DECADENT COFFEE drinks but hate the cost and extra calories of those from the coffee stores! This refreshing drink saves you money and inches from your waist." If you don't have time to brew the coffee, dissolve 2 teaspoons instant espresso in 4 ounces warm water and chill.

½ cup cold double-strength or espresso coffee

1 cup fat-free plain yogurt

1½ tablespoons agave nectar

½ cup crushed ice

TOTAL TIME: 5 MINUTES

Combine the coffee, yogurt, and nectar in a blender. Pulse to mix. Add the ice and blend for 15 seconds, or just until incorporated.

PER SERVING: 201 calories; 0 g total fat; 0 g saturated fat; 45 g carbohydrate; 0 g fiber; 10 g protein; 5 mg cholesterol; 152 mg sodium

super fast snacks

10 quick and easy snacks

two snacks daily is an important part of the 2-Week Turnaround plan. Snacks stave off hunger while keeping blood sugar in check. But you may not have the time to prepare some of these fantastic recipes every day. No problem—following are 10 super fast yet super delicious snacks to keep you on track while enjoying every bite.

The 2-Week Turnaround snack should include 200 calories made up of one dairy and one fruit. The following advice was used in the 10 simple snacks included here (each ready in minutes) and can also be used when putting together your own snacks.

CHOOSE CHEESE. A great source of both protein and calcium, portable cheese makes getting these nutrients a breeze. Be sure to go for reduced-fat or fat-free cheeses, and change them up for variety. String cheese sticks are great for on the-go snacks. Try a variety of Swiss or Cheddar types for sharpness. Often, the sharper the cheese, the more satisfying it will be. And why not do as the French do and eat the cheese with apples, pears, or grapes—a sure winner every time.

GRAB A GLASS OF MILK. Perfect for when pushed for time, a glass of fat-free milk takes care of your dairy requirement for each snack. Add a piece of fruit and you're good to go. Consider individual-size aseptic packs of milk to keep in the office or pack in the car while running errands. This way you'll always be prepared when hunger creeps up on you. And if you don't eat dairy, almond milk can provide the protein and calcium you need. Just be sure to use only unsweetened almond milk with calcium.

PICK SOME FRUIT. Fruit provides carbohydrates and fiber to ward off hunger while adding sweetness and crunch to your snack. Experiment with different kinds, reaching for what's in season. After all, don't apples taste best when freshly picked in the fall?

OPT FOR YOGURT. You'll see lots of yogurt low-fat or fat-free throughout the pages of this book. Why? It's rich and creamy, giving you that sense of comfort and decadence with every bite. Greek-style yogurt is so versatile that you can use it for a dip or salad dressing or add some agave nectar, honey, or stevia for a sweet treat. A favorite of mine is to stir in some cocoa powder and stevia!

TURKEY ROLL-UPS

This recipe makes a good pre/postworkout snack.

2 thick slices (2 ounces) reduced-
sodium fat-free deli turkey breast

1 teaspoon honey mustard

2 thin slices (1½ ounces) light
Jarlsberg cheese

½ red bell pepper, cut into thin strips

1. Lay the turkey slices on a work surface. Divide the mustard between the slices and spread over each. Top each with 1 slice of the cheese.
2. Arrange half of the pepper strips on the center of each. Roll the turkey and cheese around the peppers.

MAKES 1 SERVING

PER SERVING: 203 calories; 9 g total fat; 4 g saturated fat; 9 g carbohydrate; 2 g fiber; 25 g protein; 45 mg cholesterol; 457 mg sodium

BUFFALO CELERY STICKS

This recipe makes a good pre/postworkout snack.

4 ounces low-fat cream cheese,
softened

⅓ cup crumbled reduced-fat
blue cheese

⅛ to ¼ teaspoon hot sauce

4 ribs celery, cut into 3" pieces

Stir together the cream cheese, blue cheese, and hot sauce in a small bowl until well blended. Divide among the celery pieces.

MAKES 2 SERVINGS

PER SERVING: 172 calories; 11 g total fat; 8 g saturated fat; 7 g carbohydrate; 2 g fiber; 11 g protein; 36 mg cholesterol; 584 mg sodium

nutrition notes

◆ ANY WAY YOU *slice it, turkey breast is a lean, good-for-you protein pick. To keep your diet clean, look for nitrate-free deli turkey; nitrates are a known carcinogen.*

◆ CHEESE *is full of protein, calcium, and other essential nutrients needed for good health. But it is also loaded with calories, fat, and artery-clogging saturated fat. The best way to take advantage of cheese's good-for-you benefits without any of the bad-for-you effects is simply to choose low-fat or fat-free products.*

nutrition notes

● A RECENT STUDY *showed that people who ate three servings of yogurt per day with a lower-calorie diet lost 22 percent more weight and 61 percent more body fat than people who just cut calories. And fat-free Greek yogurt is much creamier than regular fat-free yogurt.*

● GOAT CHEESE *not only has a full, rich flavor, it is naturally lower in fat and calories than cow's milk cheese.*

GORGONZOLA DIP WITH CRUDITÉS

This recipe makes a good pre/postworkout snack.

⅓ cup crumbled Gorgonzola cheese

1 cup fat-free plain Greek-style yogurt

1 tablespoon chopped chives or scallion

2 cups assorted sliced vegetable sticks, such as carrots, peppers, and celery

Finely crumble the cheese with a large spoon in a medium bowl. Add the yogurt and chives or scallion and stir well until combined. Serve with the vegetable sticks.

MAKES 2 SERVINGS

PER SERVING: 168 calories; 6 g total fat; 4 g saturated fat; 14 g carbohydrate; 4 g fiber; 15 g protein; 17 mg cholesterol; 358 mg sodium

STUFFED ROMAINE SPEARS

This recipe makes a good pre/postworkout snack.

2 ounces low-fat goat cheese, at room temperature

Pinch of thyme or rubbed sage

½ small apple, cored and finely chopped

8 small romaine or endive leaves

1. Mash the cheese and thyme in a small bowl with a fork until smooth. Stir in the apple.

2. Arrange the leaves on a plate. Divide the cheese mixture onto the wide end of each leaf. Roll to surround the cheese with the lettuce.

MAKES 1 SERVING

PER SERVING: 157 calories; 7 g total fat; 3 g saturated fat; 16 g carbohydrate; 3 g fiber; 10 g protein; 10 mg cholesterol; 203 mg sodium

PARMESAN CHEESE CRISPS

This recipe makes a good pre/postworkout snack.

1 cup finely shredded Parmesan cheese

Freshly ground black pepper

4 small ripe pears, cut into wedges

1. Preheat the oven to 350°F. Line a large baking sheet with parchment paper or foil and coat with cooking spray. Spoon the cheese by tablespoonfuls, spacing 1″ apart, on the paper. Spread each into a 2″ round. Grind a small amount of pepper on top of each round.

2. Bake for 7 to 8 minutes, or just until golden. Quickly loosen the cheese crisps from the parchment, using a thin-bladed spatula. Cool on the pan for 5 minutes and serve with the pear wedges.

MAKES 4 SERVINGS

PER SERVING: 172 calories; 6 g total fat; 4 g saturated fat; 24 g carbohydrate; 5 g fiber; 8 g protein; 18 mg cholesterol; 307 mg sodium

MINI PESTO PIZZA

This recipe makes a good pre/postworkout snack.

½ whole grain English muffin

1 tablespoon prepared pesto

3 tablespoons shredded reduced-fat mozzarella cheese

1. Preheat the oven to broil.

2. Place the muffin upside down on a baking sheet and broil for 4 minutes, or until toasted.

3. Turn and spread with the pesto. Top with the cheese and broil for 3 minutes, or until the cheese melts.

MAKES 1 SERVING

PER SERVING: 197 calories; 11 g total fat; 4 g saturated fat; 15 g carbohydrate; 3 g fiber; 12 g protein; 16 mg cholesterol; 425 mg sodium

nutrition notes

● PEARS *are high in fiber, which can help reduce cholesterol levels—and keep you feeling full. They're also a great source of vitamins C and K and the important electrolyte potassium.*

● PESTO *is a simple sauce made from basil, olive oil, pine nuts, garlic, and Parmesan cheese. Full of healthy fats and nutrients, pesto adds a kick of taste, but be sure to use this flavorful sauce moderately to keep calories in check.*

nutrition notes

● FOODS *with a high glycemic index are digested quickly and tend to cause a spike in blood-sugar levels, making you feel hungrier faster. And according to a study in the* American Journal of Clinical Nutrition, *agave nectar's glycemic index (GI) value is about five times lower than table sugar's. Agave is also sweeter than honey, so you can use less of it.*

● DUE TO ITS MEDICINAL *properties, cinnamon has been used in many cultures for treating a variety of health disorders, including digestive problems, arthritis, menstrual issues, yeast infections, and colds.*

BLUEBERRY LEMON POPS

This recipe makes a good pre/postworkout snack.

1¾ cups fat-free plain Greek-style yogurt

1 tablespoon lemon juice

2 teaspoons agave nectar or honey

½ teaspoon lemon zest

1 cup blueberries

1. Stir together the yogurt, lemon juice, nectar or honey, and lemon zest in a medium bowl. Stir in the blueberries.

2. Divide among 2 large paper cups (about 8 ounces each). Freeze for 1 hour, or until almost set. Insert an ice-pop stick and freeze for 1 hour, or until completely set.

MAKES 2 SERVINGS

PER SERVING: 206 calories; 0 g total fat; 0 g saturated fat; 35 g carbohydrate; 2 g fiber; 18 g protein; 0 mg cholesterol; 73 mg sodium

SWEET YOGURT DIP

¾ cup fat-free plain Greek-style yogurt

1 teaspoon honey

¼ teaspoon cinnamon

Pinch of cardamom

12 caramel mini rice cakes

Stir together the yogurt, honey, cinnamon, and cardamom in a small bowl. Serve with the rice cakes for dipping.

MAKES 1 SERVING

PER SERVING: 205 calories; 3 g total fat; 0 g saturated fat; 28 g carbohydrate; 0 g fiber; 16 g protein; 0 mg cholesterol; 372 mg sodium

RASPBERRY PEACHES WITH GREEK YOGURT

This recipe makes a good pre/postworkout snack.

1 medium peach, chopped

1 tablespoon raspberry spreadable
    fruit

1 teaspoon orange juice or water

Pinch of apple pie spice

1 cup fat-free plain Greek-style yogurt

Gently stir together the peach, spreadable fruit, orange juice or water, and spice in a medium bowl until combined. Using a slotted spoon, spoon just the peaches into a dessert bowl. Top with the yogurt and drizzle with the raspberry juices.

MAKES 1 SERVING

PER SERVING: 222 calories; 1 g total fat; 0 g saturated fat; 35 g carbohydrate; 2 g fiber; 21 g protein; 0 mg cholesterol; 83 mg sodium

MELON, BERRY, AND BRIE COUPE

This recipe makes a good pre/postworkout snack.

½ cup chopped cantaloupe

½ cup quartered strawberries

¼ cup cubed Brie

¼ to ½ teaspoon aged balsamic
    vinegar

Stir together the cantaloupe, strawberries, and Brie in a small bowl. Drizzle with the balsamic vinegar.

MAKES 1 SERVING

PER SERVING: 173 calories; 10 g total fat; 6 g saturated fat; 13 g carbohydrate; 2 g fiber; 9 g protein; 36 mg cholesterol; 240 mg sodium

nutrition notes

▸ A FEW YEARS AGO, *the nonprofit Environmental Working Group ranked 43 commonly consumed fruits and vegetables using "total pesticide load" results collected by the USDA and the FDA. Peaches ranked as the number one most-contaminated fruit. To help reduce your exposure to potentially harmful chemicals, buy organic peaches whenever possible.*

▸ STRAWBERRIES, *as well as blueberries, raspberries, and blackberries, are rich in compounds called phenols, which have antioxidant properties and can help protect against cancer and heart disease.*

CHAPTER 7 ∘ SNACKS AND DESSERTS

appendix

The 2-Week Total Body Turnaround Jump-Start Routine

If you've already tried the 2-Week Total Body Turnaround plan, you know that the secret to success lies in the program's slow-motion strength routine. Instead of lifting and lowering for 2 counts each, you'll double the lengthening "eccentric" phase of an exercise (i.e., straightening your arm during a biceps curl) to 4 counts. "In eccentric training, each muscle fiber works harder so you get firmer faster," explains Freytag. An East Carolina University study found that, after just 1 week, women who did eccentric training increased their strength by nearly twice as much as those who lifted weights at a normal pace. You'll also build more muscle and rev up your metabolism to burn fat faster.

As you've seen in the stories throughout the book, when we put a group of readers on the plan, the results were eye-popping: Testers lost an average of 6 pounds and 10 inches in 14 days, with the most successful volunteers losing up to 12 pounds and more than 22 inches all over.

If you haven't tried the plan yet, get started today with this abbreviated jump-start routine. Adapted from the original program, it will help you shed pounds, lose inches, and feel confident in just 14 days! And for more super-effective strength exercises and cardio routines that work superfast, pick up a copy of *2-Week Total Body Turnaround*.

YOUR 2-WEEK TURNAROUND	
Day 1	Strength Plan A; Speed Ladder
Day 2	Strength Plan B; Power Walk
Day 3	Strength Plan A; Speed Ladder
Day 4	Strength Plan B; Power Walk
Day 5	Strength Plan A; Speed Ladder
Day 6	Strength Plan B; Power Walk
Day 7	**Active rest (no formal workout, but keep moving throughout the day)**
Day 8	Strength Plan A with Make It Harder options; Speed Ladder
Day 9	Strength Plan B with Make It Harder options; Power Walk
Day 10	Strength Plan A with Make It Harder options; Speed Ladder
Day 11	**Active rest**
Day 12	Strength Plan B with Make It Harder options; Power Walk
Day 13	Strength Plan A with Make It Harder options; Speed Ladder
Day 14	Strength Plan B with Make It Harder options; Power Walk

For continued success, repeat or modify to alternate cardio and strength workouts.

Adapted from 2-Week Total Body Turnaround by Chris Freytag with Alyssa Shaffer and the editors of Prevention (Rodale, 2009).

THE STRENGTH PLAN WORKOUT **A**

1. HIP DROP | TARGETS: *Abs, obliques*

A. Lie face down on the floor, with your legs extended, and your elbows and forearms on the floor. Lift your hips, keeping abs tight while forming a straight line from your head to your heels.

B. Tip slightly to the right, keeping your back straight, as you lower your right hip to the floor in 4 counts. Return to the start position in 2 counts. Tip toward your left side for 4 counts. Come back to the start position in 2 counts. Continue for 8 to 10 repetitions on each side.

Make It Harder (Week 2): Do 12 to 15 times each side.

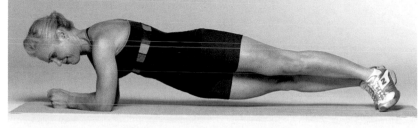

2. BEACH BALL HUG | TARGETS: *Chest, abs, hips*

A. Lie face up on the floor, with your knees bent and your feet flat on the floor. Hold dumbbells above your chest with your arms extended, elbows slightly bent, and palms facing each other. Lift your left leg, keeping your knee bent 90 degrees, and your shin parallel to the floor.

B. Slowly lower your arms out to sides in 4 counts, keeping your elbows slightly bent while simultaneously "reaching" your left foot out to straighten your leg. Pull your knee back to the start position in 2 counts while lifting your arms back above your chest, squeezing your chest muscles as if you're hugging a beach ball. Repeat 6 times with your left leg, then do the exercise 6 times with your right leg.

Make It Harder (Week 2): Raise both feet off floor.

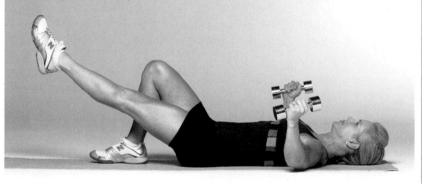

WORKOUT AT A GLANCE

THE STRENGTH PLAN

What you'll need: 2 sets of dumbbells (2 to 5 and 8 to 10 pounds); a chair.

Week 1: Do the routine 6 days a week, alternating between Workout A (for your chest, back, and abs) and Workout B (for your arms, legs, and butt).

Week 2: Follow the same schedule, but challenge yourself by trying the Make It Harder options.

THE CARDIO PLAN

Weeks 1 & 2: Walk for 30 minutes 6 days a week, alternating between the Speed Ladder interval routine and Power Walk workout (page 257).

3. FULL-BODY ROLL-UP | TARGETS: *Abs*

A. Lie face up on the floor, with your legs slightly bent and your arms extended next to your head, and your shoulders relaxed, palms facing each other. Pressing your shoulders down, slowly roll up off the floor in 4 counts, keeping your abs pulled in and your arms extended.

B. Finish by reaching forward toward your toes. Slowly roll back down to the floor to the starting position, taking about 6 to 8 counts to lower. Repeat 6 to 8 times.

Make It Harder (Week 2): Hold a light weight (2 to 3 pounds) in both hands.

GOOD FORM TIP:
Keep your heels on the mat as you roll up; use just your abs to move you up, not your hip flexors.

4. BREAST STROKE | TARGETS: *Upper and middle back*

A. Lie face down on the floor, with your arms extended overhead and your palms facing each other. Lift your head and arms off the floor, keeping your abs tight and your head in line with your spine. Hold here for 2 counts.

B. Lift your chest a few inches off the floor and "swim" your arms down in 2 counts, sweeping them out in semicircles toward the middle of your back. (Finish with your thumbs pointing down,) Use the middle back muscles to keep you up. Be sure to keep your abs tight and your feet on the floor. As you lower your chest, draw your arms in toward your body, bending your elbows, then "swim" them back overhead to the start position in 4 counts. Do 8 to 10 reps.

Make It Harder (Week 2): As you lift your chest and swim your arms, raise both feet off floor, then lower.

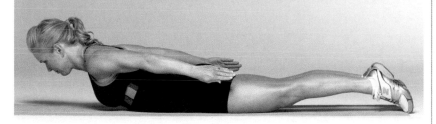

5. READ THE PAPER | TARGETS: *Abs, obliques*

A. Sit on the floor with your knees bent and your heels on floor. Hold your arms in front of your body, as if holding a closed newspaper.

B. Slowly lower your upper body toward the floor, rounding your back. Stop about halfway down, and twist to your left, as if opening the paper on your left side, in 4 counts. With a big exhale, take 2 counts and pull yourself back to the start position, using your obliques (the muscles in the sides of your torso). Repeat on the right side. Do 8 to 12 times total.

Make It Harder (Week 2): Hold a light weight (2 to 3 pounds) in each hand.

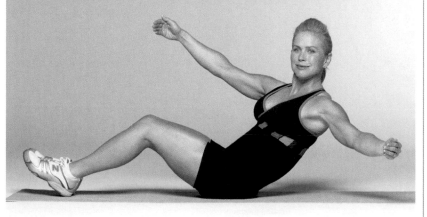

THE STRENGTH PLAN WORKOUT B

1. PLIÉ WITH BICEPS CURL

TARGETS: *Biceps, butt, quads, inner thighs*

A. Stand with your feet shoulder-width apart, toes turned outward, holding dumbbells in front of your thighs with palms facing up.

B. Slowly lower your body straight down for 2 counts, bending your knees 90 degrees while simultaneously curling weights toward your shoulders. Slowly stand back up for 4 counts, squeezing your butt and inner thighs, as you lower your arms back to the starting position. Repeat 8 to 12 times.

Make It Harder (Week 2): Use heavier weights.

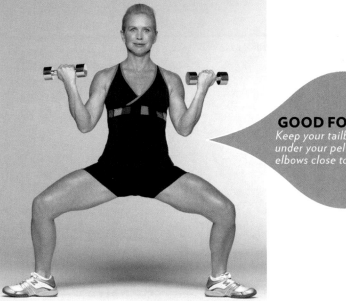

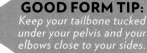

GOOD FORM TIP: *Keep your tailbone tucked under your pelvis and your elbows close to your sides.*

2. FORWARD LUNGE AND RAISE THE ROOF

TARGETS: *Shoulders, quads, butt, core*

A. Stand with your feet together, holding dumbbells overhead, palms facing forward.

B. Lunge forward with your right foot in 4 counts, bending both knees 90 degrees while lowering weights toward your shoulders, by bending your elbows 90 degrees. Push back to starting the position and straighten your arms in 2 counts. Repeat 8 to 12 times; switch sides.

Make It Harder (Week 2): Swing your left knee forward to hip height as you stand up.

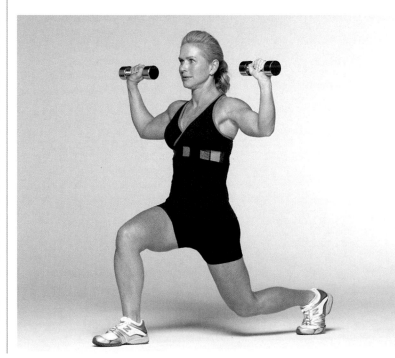

3. SQUAT WITH STRAIGHT-ARM PRESSBACK

TARGETS: *Shoulders, arms, quads, butt*

A. Stand with your feet about 4 inches apart, holding dumbbells at your sides with palms facing behind you. Slowly lower into squat position for 4 counts, keeping body weight over your heels your as your arms move forward.

B. Stand back up in 2 counts while pressing your palms behind you. Repeat 8 to 12 times.

Make It Harder (Week 2): Lift your left leg back and squeeze your glutes as you stand; switch legs halfway through the set.

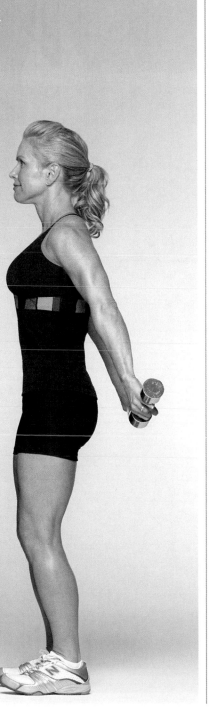

4. CURTSY LAT RAISE

TARGETS: *Shoulders, butt, quads, outer thighs*

A. Stand with your feet shoulder-width apart, holding dumbbells at your sides. Cross your right leg 2 to 3 feet behind your left, bending your knees. At the same time, lift your right arm out to the side at shoulder height. Take 4 counts to perform.

B. Stand up in 2 counts, bringing your right leg back to the starting position as you lower your arm. Repeat 8 times. Switch sides, repeat 8 times.

Make It Harder (Week 2): As you stand up, lift your right leg out to the side.

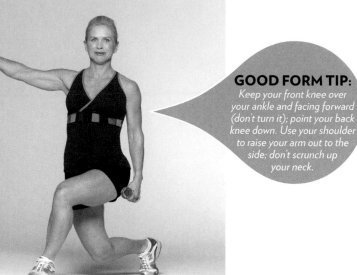

GOOD FORM TIP: *Keep your front knee over your ankle and facing forward (don't turn it); point your back knee down. Use your shoulder to raise your arm out to the side; don't scrunch up your neck.*

5. TIP IT OVER

TARGETS: *Arms, shoulders, hamstrings, butt*

A. Start with your feet staggered, right foot in front of left. Hold a dumbbell in your left hand while holding the back of a chair or seat with your right hand. Keeping your spine straight and your abs tight, lean forward in 4 counts. Reach your left arm toward the floor while lifting your left leg behind you, slightly softening your knee.

B. Return to the start position in 2 counts, curling the weight toward your shoulder in a biceps curl while lifting your left knee to hip height.

C. Slowly press the weight up toward the ceiling in 2 counts and lower it in 4 counts. Repeat 8 times, then switch sides.

Make It Harder (Week 2): Use a heavier weight and skip the chair.

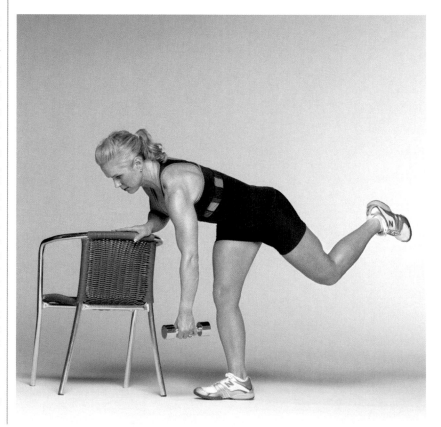

THE CARDIO PLANS

SPEED LADDER

This challenging workout features intervals that get increasingly harder but shorter, followed by brief recovery periods.

TIME	ACTIVITY (SPEED*)	INTENSITY**	HOW IT FEELS
0:00	Warm-up (3.0 MPH)	4	Breathing harder; can speak in full sentences
4:00	Moderate walk (3.5 MPH)	5	Slightly breathless; can still speak in full sentences
9:00	Brisk walk (3.75 MPH)	6	Somewhat breathless; can speak in short sentences only
13:00	Moderate walk (3.5 MPH)	5	
15:00	Power walk (4.0 MPH)	7	Mostly breathless; can speak in phrases only
18:00	Moderate walk (3.5 MPH)	5	
20:00	Fast walk (4.5 MPH)	8	Breathless; can speak just a few words at a time
22:00	Moderate walk (3.5 MPH)	5	
24:00	Speed walk or jog (5.0 MPH)	9	Very breathless; can't speak
25:00	Cool down (3.0 MPH)	4	Breathing slows
30:00	Finished		

*These are suggested speeds only and may not be appropriate for everyone. The right speed for you should be based on intensity recommendations and how you feel.

**Based on a 1-to-10 scale, with 1 being extremely easy and 10 so hard that you can't sustain the pace for more than a few seconds.

POWER WALK

This cardio routine is a great way to build endurance while burning calories.

TIME	ACTIVITY (SPEED*)	INTENSITY**	HOW IT FEELS
0:00	Warm-up (3.0 MPH)	4	Breathing harder; can speak in full sentences
5:00	Power walk (3.5–4.0 MPH)	5–7	Somewhat breathless; can speak in short sentences only
25:00	Cool down (3.0 MPH)	4	Breathing slows
30:00	Finished		

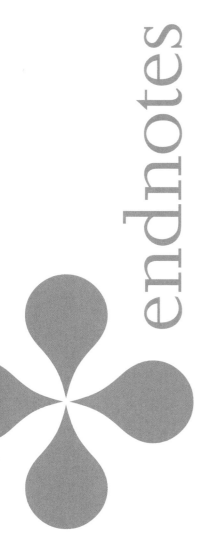

endnotes

CHAPTER 1

1 T.R. Kirk and M.C. Cursiter, "Long-term snacking intervention did not lead to weight gain in free-living man," *Scandinavian Journal of Nutrition* 2(1999):3-17.

2 H. Yates, N.E. Crombie, and T.R. Kirk, "Evidence of energy intake compensation at meals after snacking intervention—a pilot study," *International Journal on Obesity*, 21(1997):S113.

3 "Is eating between meals good for our health?" European Food Information Council, www.eufic.org/article/en/page/RARCHIVE/expid/review-eating-between-meals-health (accessed on 9/23/09).

4 "Eating and exercise: Time it right to maximize your workout," Mayo Clinic, www.mayoclinic.com/health/exercise/HQ00594_D (accessed on 9/23/09).

5 K.M. Zawadzki, B.B. Yaspelkis, and J.L. Ivy, "Carbohydrate-protein complex increases the rate of muscle glycogen storage after exercise," *Journal of Applied Physiology* 72(1992):1854–1859.

6 "Eating and exercise: Time it right to maximize your workout," Mayo Clinic, www.mayoclinic.com/health/exercise/HQ00594_D (accessed on 9/23/09).

7 "Metabolism and weight loss: How you burn calories," Mayo Clinic, www.mayoclinic.com/health/metabolism/WT00006 (accessed on 9/24/09).

8 "Fatigue fighters—six quick ways to boost energy," WebMD, http://women.webmd.com/features/fatigue-fighters-six-quick-ways-boost-energy (accessed on 9/23/09).

9 "10 ways to boost your metabolism," WebMD, www.webmd.com/diet/slideshow-boost-your-metabolism (accessed on 9/23/09).

10 T.L. Halton and F.B. Hu, "The effects of high protein diets on thermogenesis, satiety, and weight loss: a critical review," *Journal of the American College of Nutrition*, 23 no.5 (2004):373-385.

CHAPTER 2

1 M. Noakes, J.B. Keogh, P.R. Foster, and P.M. Clifton, "Effect of an energy-restricted, high-protein, low-fat diet relative to a conventional high-carbohydrate, high-fat diet on weight loss, body composition, nutritional status, and markers of cardiovascular health in obese women," *American Journal of Clinical Nutrition*, 81 no. 6 (2005):1298-1306.

2 T. McLaughlin, S. Carter, C. Lamendola et al, "Effects of moderate variations in macronutrient compositions on weight loss and reduction in cardiovascular disease risk in obese, insulin-resistant adults," *American Journal of Clinical Nutrition*, 84 no. 4(2006):813-821.

3 "Fruit & vegetable benefits," Centers for Disease Control and Prevention, www.fruitsandveggiesmatter.gov/benefits/index.html (accessed on 9/23/09).

4 "Phytochemicals," Dole 5 A Day Reference Center, http://216.255.136.121/ReferenceCenter/NutritionCenter/Phytochemicals/pdf/index.jsp?topmenu=1 (accessed on 9/23/09).

5 "Phytochemicals," Linus Pauling Institute, http://lpi.oregonstate.edu/infocenter/phytochemicals.html (accessed on 9/23/09).

6 "Antioxidants," MedlinePlus, www.nlm.nih.gov/medlineplus/antioxidants.html (accessed on 9/23/09).

7 L. Packer, E. Cadenas, and K.J.A. Davies, "Free radicals and exercise: an introduction," *Free Radical Biology & Medicine*, 44 no. 2 (2008):123-125.

8 "Food sources the best choices for antioxidants," Mayo Clinic www.mayoclinic.org/medical-edge-newspaper-2009/jun-05b.html (accessed on 9/23/09).

9 "Low-carb diets: the right way to go?" University of Maryland Medical Center, www.umm.edu/features/low_carb_diets.htm (accessed on 9/23/09).

10 "Whole grains: Hearty options for a healthy diet," Mayo Clinic, www. mayoclinic.com/health/whole-grains/NU00204 (accessed on 9/23/09).

11 "Health gains from whole grains," Harvard School of Public Health, www. hsph.harvard.edu/nutritionsource/what-should-you-eat/health-gains-from-whole-grains/index.html (accessed on 9/23/09).

12 "Whole grains fact sheet," International Food Information Council, www.ific.org/publications/factsheets/wholegrainsfs.cfm (accessed on 9/23/09).

13 S. Liu, W.C. Willett, J.E. Manson, F.B. Hu, B. Rosner, and G. Colditz, "Relation between changes in intakes of dietary fiber and grain products and changes in weight and development of obesity among middle-aged women," *American Journal of Clinical Nutrition*, 78(2003):920-927.

14 P. Koh-Banerjee, M. Franz, L. Sampson, S. Liu, D.R.J. Jacobs, D. Spiegelman, W. Willett, and E. Rimm, "Changes in whole-grain, bran, and cereal fiber consumption in relation to 8-y weight gain among men," *American Journal of Clinical Nutrition*, 80(2004):1237-45.

15 "Calcium and bone health," Centers for Disease Control and Prevention, www.cdc.gov/nutrition/everyone/basics/vitamins/calcium.html (accessed on 9/23/09).

16 "Calcium and bone health," Centers for Disease Control and Prevention, www.cdc.gov/nutrition/everyone/basics/vitamins/calcium.html (accessed on 9/23/09).

17 "Fasts facts on osteoporosis," National Osteoporosis Foundation, www. nof.org/osteoporosis/diseasefacts.htm (accessed on 9/23/09).

18 "Osteoporosis bone health," National Osteoporosis Foundation, www.nof. org/osteoporosis/bonehealth.htm (accessed on 9/23/09).

19 "Fasts facts on osteoporosis," National Osteoporosis Foundation, www. nof.org/osteoporosis/diseasefacts.htm (accessed on 9/23/09).

20 L. Wang, J.E. Manson, J.E. Buring, I. Lee, and H.D. Sesso, "Dietary intake of dairy products, calcium, and vitamin D and the risk of hypertension in middle-aged and older women," *Hypertension*, 51(2008):1073-1079.

21 M.B. Zemel, W. Thompson, A. Milstead et al, "Calcium and dairy acceleration of weight and fat loss during energy restriction in obese adults," *Obesity Research*, 12 no. 4 (2004):582-590.

22 E.L. Melanson, W.T. Donahoo, F. Dong, T. Ida, and M.B. Zemel, "Effect of low- and high-calcium dairy-based diets on macronutrient oxidation in humans," *Obesity Research*, 13(2005):2102-12.

23 A.J. Lanou and N.D. Barnard, "Dairy and weight loss hypothesis: an evaluation of the clinical trials," *Nutrition Review*, 66 no. 5 (2008):272-279.

ENDNOTES

24 "Calcium and bone health," Centers for Disease Control and Prevention, www.cdc.gov/nutrition/everyone/basics/vitamins/calcium.html (accessed on 9/23/09).

25 "Protein: Moving closer to center stage," Harvard School of Public Health, www.hsph.harvard.edu/nutritionsource/what-should-you-eat/protein-full-story/index.html#introduction (accessed on 9/23/09).

26 "Can one change improve your health and the world's?" Mayo Clinic, www.mayoclinic.com/health/red-meat/MY00788 (accessed on 9/23/09).

27 "Saturated fat," Centers for Disease Control and Prevention, www.cdc.gov/nutrition/everyone/basics/fat/saturatedfat.html (accessed on 9/23/09).

28 "Trans fat," Centers for Disease Control and Prevention, www.cdc.gov/nutrition/everyone/basics/fat/transfat.html (accessed on 9/23/09).

29 B.M. Davy, E.A. Dennis, A.L. Dengo et al, "Water consumption reduces energy intake at a breakfast meal in obese older adults," *Journal of the American Dietetic Association*, 108 no. 7 (2008):1236-1239.

30 M. Boschmann, J. Steiniger, U. Hille et al, "Water-induced thermogenesis," *Journal of Clinical Endocrinology & Metabolism*, 88 no. 12 (2003):6015-6019.

31 "Eating and exercise: Time it right to maximize your workout," Mayo Clinic, http://mayoclinic.com/health/exercise/HQ00594_D/NSECTIONGROUP=2 (accessed on 9/23/09).

CHAPTER 3

1 A. A. Gorin, H.A. Raynor, H.M. Niemeier, and R.R. Wing, "Home grocery delivery improves the household food environments of behavioral weight loss participants: results of an 8-week pilot study," *International Journal of Behavioral Nutrition and Physical Activity*, 4(2007):58.

2 "Trans fat is double trouble for your heart health," Mayo Clinic, www.mayoclinic.com/health/trans-fat/CL00032 (accessed on 9/23/09).

3 "Top 10 healthy cooking tips," American Heart Association, www.americanheart.org/presenter.jhtml?identifier=3039951 (accessed on 9/23/09).

4 "Sodium: Are you getting too much?" Mayo Clinic, www.mayoclinic.com/health/sodium/NU00284 (accessed on 9/23/09).

5 "Eat local: Does your food travel more than you do?" Natural Resources Defense Council, www.nrdc.org/health/foodmiles (accessed on 9/23/09).

6 "Healthy eating," AFB Senior Site, www.afb.org/seniorsite.asp?SectionID=63&TopicID=396&DocumentID=4229 (accessed on 9/23/09).

7 N.I. Larson, D. Neumark-Sztainer, P.J. Hannan, and M. Story, "Family meals during adolescence are associated with higher diet quality and healthful meal patterns during young adulthood," *Journal of the American Dietetic Association*, 107 no. 9(2007):1502-1510.

8 "Carbohydrate-loading diet," Mayo Clinic, www.mayoclinic.com/health/carbohydrate-loading/MY00223 (accessed on 9/23/09).

CHAPTER 4

1 K. Fujioka et al, "The effects of grapefruit on weight and insulin resistance: relationship to the metabolic syndrome," *Journal of Medicinal Food*, 9(2006):49-54.

2 K.J. Acheson et al, "Caffeine and coffee: their influence on metabolic rate and substrate oxidation in normal weight and obese individuals," *American Journal of Clinical Nutrition*, 33(1980):989-997.

3 M.S. Westerterp-Plantenga, et al., "Body weight loss and weight maintenance in relation to habitual caffeine intake and green tea supplementation," *Obesity Research*, 13(2005):1195-1204.

CHAPTER 5

1 "Green tea," University of Maryland Medical Center, www.umm.edu/altmed/articles/green-tea-000255.htm (accessed on 9/23/09).

2 K. Diepvens et al, "Obesity and thermogenesis related to the consumption of caffeine, ephedrine, capsaicin, and green tea," *American Journal of Physiology–Regulatory, Intergrative and Comparative Physiology*, 292(2007):R77-R85.

3 S. Berube-Parent et al, "Effects of encapsulated green tea and Guarana extracts containing a mixture of epigallocatechin-3-gallate and caffeine on 24 h energy expenditure and fat oxidation in men," *British Journal of Nutrition*, 94(2005):432-436.

4 "Whole grains fact sheet," International Food Information Council, www.ific.org/publications/factsheets/wholegrainsfs.cfm#Finding%20Whole%20Grain%20Foods (accessed on 10/19/09).

CHAPTER 6

1 M. Yoshioka et al, "Effects of red pepper added to high-fat and high-carbohydrate meals on energy metabolism and substrate utilization in Japanese women," *British Journal of Nutrition*, 80(1998):503-510.

2 M.S. Westerterp-Plantenga, A. Smeets, and M.P.G Lejeune, "Sensory and gastrointestinal satiety effects of capsaicin on food intake," *International Journal of Obesity*, 29(2005):682-688.

CHAPTER 7

1 M. Van Loan. "The role of dairy foods and dietary calcium in weight management," *Journal of the American College of Nutrition*, 28(2009):120S-129S.

2 "Calcium: Drink yourself skinny," WebMD, www.webmd.com/diet/features/calcium-weight-loss (accessed on 9/23/09).

index

Underscored page references indicate boxed text. **Boldfaced** page references indicate photographs.

CONVERSION CHART

These equivalents have been slightly rounded to make measuring easier.

VOLUME MEASUREMENTS		
U.S.	IMPERIAL	METRIC
¼ tsp	–	1 ml
½ tsp	–	2 ml
1 tsp	–	5 ml
1 Tbsp	–	15 ml
2 Tbsp (1 oz)	1 fl oz	30 ml
¼ cup (2 oz)	2 fl oz	60 ml
⅓ cup (3 oz)	3 fl oz	80 ml
½ cup (4 oz)	4 fl oz	120 ml
⅔ cup (5 oz)	5 fl oz	160 ml
¾ cup (6 oz)	6 fl oz	180 ml
1 cup (8 oz)	8 fl oz	240 ml

WEIGHT MEASUREMENTS	
U.S.	METRIC
1 oz	30 g
2 oz	60 g
4 oz (¼ lb)	115 g
5 oz (⅓ lb)	145 g
6 oz	170 g
7 oz	200 g
8 oz (½ lb)	230 g
10 oz	285 g
12 oz (¾ lb)	340 g
14 oz	400 g
16 oz (1 lb)	455 g
2.2 lb	1 kg

LENGTH MEASUREMENTS	
U.S.	METRIC
¼"	0.6 cm
½"	1.25 cm
1"	2.5 cm
2"	5 cm
4"	11 cm
6"	15 cm
8"	20 cm
10"	25 cm
12" (1')	30 cm

PAN SIZES	
U.S.	METRIC
8" cake pan	20 × 4 cm sandwich or cake tin
9" cake pan	23 × 3.5 cm sandwich or cake tin
11" × 7" baking pan	28 × 18 cm baking tin
13" × 9" baking pan	32.5 × 23 cm baking tin
15" × 10" baking pan	38 × 25.5 cm baking tin (Swiss roll tin)
1½ qt baking dish	1.5 liter baking dish
2 qt baking dish	2 liter baking dish
2 qt rectangular baking dish	30 × 19 cm baking dish
9" pie plate	22 × 4 or 23 × 4 cm pie plate
7" or 8" springform pan	18 or 20 cm springform or loose-bottom cake tin
9" × 5" loaf pan	23 × 13 cm or 2 lb narrow loaf tin or pâté tin

TEMPERATURES		
FAHRENHEIT	CENTIGRADE	GAS
140°	60°	–
160°	70°	–
180°	80°	–
225°	105°	¼
250°	120°	½
275°	135°	1
300°	150°	2
325°	160°	3
350°	180°	4
375°	190°	5
400°	200°	6
425°	220°	7
450°	230°	8
475°	245°	9
500°	260°	–

about the authors

HEATHER K. JONES is a registered dietitian and author of *What's Your Diet Type?* and *The Grocery Cart Makeover*. In addition, Heather is an accomplished freelance health journalist with numerous articles published in healthy-living magazines with national circulations, and a nutrition consultant for *The Best Life Diet* by Bob Greene, Oprah's personal trainer. She also has more than 7 years' experience working for the acclaimed *Nutrition Action Healthletter,* published by the Center for Science in the Public Interest (CSPI).

CHRIS FREYTAG, a fitness professional and mother of three teenagers, understands firsthand the challenges of balancing healthy habits with the demands of a busy life. A contributing editor at *Prevention* magazine and author of *Shortcuts to Big Weight Loss,* Chris is also the founder of Motivating Bodies, Inc., a fitness coaching program. She has hosted many Prevention Fitness Systems' DVDs, is on the board of directors for the American Council on Exercise, teaches classes part-time at Life-Time Fitness, and is frequently featured in many magazines, newspapers, and TV shows.

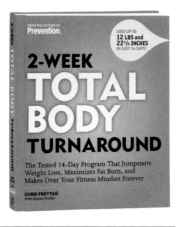
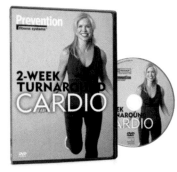
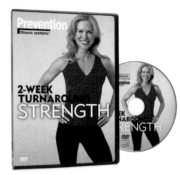